100

Ways to
Live to 100

■

77 Ways to Beat Colds and Flu

■

67 Ways to Good Sleep

■

Backache: 51 Ways to Relieve the Pain

■

Headaches: 47 Ways to Stop the Pain

■

Skin: Head-to-Toe Tips for Health and Beauty

■

Stress: 63 Ways to Relieve Tension and Stay Healthy

100
Ways to
Live to 100

■

Charles B. Inlander
and
Christine Kuehn Kelly

A *People's Medical Society* Book

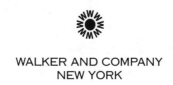

WALKER AND COMPANY
NEW YORK

A note to the reader: The ideas, procedures, and suggestions contained in this book are not intended as a substitute for consulting with your practitioner. All matters regarding your health require medical supervision.

Many of the designations used by manufacturers and sellers to distinguish their products are claimed as trademarks. Where those designations appear in this book and the authors were aware of a trademark claim, the designations have been printed with initial capital letters.

First published in the United States of America in 1999 by Walker Publishing Company, Inc.

Published simultaneously in Canada by Fitzhenry and Whiteside, Markham, Ontario, L3R 4T8

Library of Congress Cataloging-in-Publication Data

Inlander, Charles B.
100 ways to live to 100 /
Charles B. Inlander and Christine Kuehn Kelly.
p. cm.
ISBN 0-8027-7557-8 (pbk.)
1. Longevity. 2. Aged–Health and hygiene. I. Kelly, Christine Kuehn.
II. Title. III. Title: One hundred ways to live to one hundred.
RA776.75.I54 1999
613'.0438–dc21

99-17896
CIP

Printed in the United States of America

2 4 6 8 10 9 7 5 3 1

■ CONTENTS

■ PREFACE

My grandfather, born in the 1880s, lived to be 74. That was about 30 years longer than was expected at his time of birth. My father, born in 1909, turns 90 this year. He's already surpassed his birth-time life expectancy by almost 40 years. And if I live 40 years beyond what was expected in 1946, the year of my birth, I'll make it well past 100!

The reasons that my grandparents and my parents lived longer than originally calculated had a lot to do with advances in public health and medications. Yet the reasons that I—and those born after me—may live longer have more to do with lifestyle. In the last two to three decades, researchers have discovered that individual choices about what we eat, how fit we are, and how conscientious we are about safety are vital ingredients to longevity.

And that's why we have written this book. You can play a major role in how long you live. The more you know about lifestyles and activities that can shorten your life, the more likely you are to avoid them—or at least take precautions to lessen their impact. By the same token, the more you know about lifestyles and activities that can lengthen your life, the more likely you are to incorporate them into your daily routine.

Back in 1992, I coauthored the original edition of *100 Ways to Live to 100*, a very successful book. People from all over the world have told me that what we wrote helped them immensely. And they asked me to write another edition when we learned more. Well, this is it.

So much new research on living long has come forth in the past seven years. From automobile safety devices to the role of vitamins and minerals, literally hundreds of new pieces of information are available to help guide you to living a longer and healthier life. You'll find all that information in the pages that follow.

But before you start, let me explain something about this book. You'll notice we didn't number the tips. That's because we realized that there are a lot more than 100 ways to live to 100 found in these pages. So instead of trying to be cute and squeeze more than 100 tips into 100 different numbered items, we decided that in the interest of stress reduction (which, by the way, is a major factor in living longer), we would not number every tidbit of information. As a result, we've probably added a few months, if not years, to our own lives, and we've given you the bonus of *more* than 100 ways to live to 100!

Finally, for the People's Medical Society, books like this are a labor of love. Our goal since our founding in 1983 has been to empower health care consumers by passing along useful health and medical information. This book is a prime example of that mission.

Charles B. Inlander, President
People's Medical Society

■ INTRODUCTION

If you had been born 100 years ago, your average life expectancy would have been about 47 years. Today, a baby born in the United States can expect to live about 76 years. Some 3 million Americans are estimated to have celebrated their 85th birthdays in 1998, making them the fastest growing segment of our population. And about 70,000 Americans have already celebrated their 100th birthdays. By the year 2050, it's estimated that there will be at least 1 million centenarians.

Many things have contributed to this increase in life span. Improved sanitation has virtually eliminated water-borne diseases. Immunizations now protect us from viruses that once killed entire families. Safety measures such as smoke detectors and automobile seat belts save countless lives. New diagnostic procedures and medications help identify and fight deadly diseases sooner and more effectively. The genetic basis of many hereditary life-threatening diseases is being uncovered, and therapies are being developed. And an emphasis on a healthy lifestyle is helping propel people off of the couch and away from dangerous fatty foods and empty calories.

We now know that the key to successful aging lies as much in our lifestyles as in our genes. The landmark Nurses' Health Study, for example, showed that a low-fat diet, regular exercise, and a low body mass index are major determinants of how long people live. And a study of University of Pennsylvania alumni found that those who didn't smoke and who controlled their weight and exercised throughout middle and late adulthood were more likely to live longer.

But much remains to be done. Although we know about the benefits of a low-fat diet, exercise, and proper medications, heart disease continues to kill more than 960,000 Americans annually. Despite our knowledge of the effects of tobacco, lung cancer remains the leading cause of death from cancer; it killed more than 160,600 people in 1998. Colorectal cancer (cancer of the colon and/or rectum), which in many cases can be avoided by proper diet and exercise, accounted for 56,500 deaths in 1998. And prostate cancer and breast cancer each kill about 40,000 people every year, despite screening methods that can detect these diseases before they start their deadly spread.

Accidents also take their toll. In 1997, more than 42,000 people lost their lives in vehicular accidents, according to the National Highway Traffic Safety Administration. Falls are the second leading cause of preventable death in the United States. Approximately 5,000 people over the age of 75 die of fall-related complications every year, mostly in their homes. Every year, fires in the home kill another 4,000 Americans. And about 900 Americans are killed in bicycle accidents.

One important link exists in the lives cut short from these kinds of diseases and accidents: Behavioral changes could have prevented many of the deaths. And most of the changes are relatively simple. Smoking cessation is the single most important lifestyle change that can increase longevity. Other lifestyle changes, especially an emphasis on daily exercise and a diet high in fruit, vegetables, and grains, can also make an important difference in preventing diseases. Safety precautions are also likely to extend your life.

Studies also show that nonmedical factors such as spirituality, relationships, an active mind, and stress reduction—even pet ownership—are powerfully linked to living long and staying well.

Reaching the age of 100 in good mental and physical health is becoming a reality for some and a goal for many more. It makes sense, then, to take a lifelong approach to good health. The following tips, compiled from the best research on the areas that are most likely to impact longevity, will help you do just that.

1 ■ Preventing and Managing Medical Conditions

Every year, chronic diseases claim the lives of more than 1.7 million Americans. Yet many of these deaths can be prevented. The major chronic disease killers—heart disease, cancer, stroke, chronic obstructive pulmonary disease, and diabetes—are often directly related to how individuals behave in their daily lives. In other words, you can do plenty to prevent them from shortening your life. But first, you need to know something about them.

Cardiovascular diseases are the nation's leading killers. Diseases of the heart and blood vessels claim nearly 1 million lives annually. Approximately one-third of those people die prematurely—younger than their average life expectancy. Among the most common cardiovascular diseases are coronary artery disease, the leading cause of death; stroke, the third leading cause of death; and hypertension (high blood pressure), which contributes to death from both heart attack and stroke.

Coronary artery disease and most strokes are largely the result of atherosclerosis, a buildup of fat, cholesterol, and other substances on the inside of artery walls. As the walls become lined with layers of these deposits, known as plaque, the arteries narrow, reducing the flow of blood—and oxygen—to the body. When atherosclerosis affects the coronary arteries, which supply blood to the heart, the resulting

1

oxygen deficiency can produce the chest pain known as angina pectoris. If blood flow is severely reduced or blocked, perhaps by a blood clot, the result is a heart attack, in which a portion of the heart muscle literally starves to death. Likewise, a blockage of the carotid arteries, which supply blood to the brain, can lead to stroke—the oxygen-starvation death of an area of the brain.

Although heart disease is the nation's number one killer, more people fear the number two killer—cancer. An estimated 8 million Americans are alive today who have cancer or are cancer survivors, but the disease remains deadly for many. It killed an estimated 564,800 Americans in 1998. Of the more than 100 types of cancer, lung, breast, and colorectal cancers are the deadliest for women. For men, lung, prostate, and colorectal cancers are the deadliest.

Chronic bronchitis may not sound that dangerous, but along with emphysema, it is the fourth leading cause of death in the United States. Collectively known as chronic obstructive pulmonary disease (COPD), the conditions block the flow of air out of the bronchial passages, affecting the body's ability to get oxygen. In chronic bronchitis, the blockage is caused by persistent inflammation of the lining of the bronchial passages; in emphysema, it's caused by enlargement of the air sacs in the lungs. COPD killed an estimated 106,146 Americans in 1996. And the incidence of the disease has increased 60 percent since 1982.

Diabetes is the seventh leading cause of death, according the National Center for Health Statistics. It directly caused 61,559 deaths in 1996 and contributed to nearly three times that many. Diabetes is a breakdown of the body's ability to use the hormone insulin, which enables cells to absorb glucose (blood sugar) for use as energy. In type 1 diabetes, the body virtually stops producing insulin. In type 2 diabetes, the more common form, the cells become resistant to the effects of insulin. In either case, high levels of glucose in the blood result.

High blood glucose levels cause the kidneys to work overtime. And the shortage of sugar causes the body's cells to use protein and fat for energy. The breakdown of these fats releases toxic acids called ketones, which can poison the body. All in all, diabetes hastens wear and tear on many crucial bodily functions. Left unchecked, diabetes can lead to dangerous complications such as heart disease, stroke, circulation problems, and kidney failure.

In this chapter, we offer an overview of the causes and risk factors for the major illnesses that can shorten your life, along with a summary of the steps you can take to reduce your risks. And for those times that risk reduction isn't enough, we tell you how to get the very best medical care–care that can extend your life.

 ## Determine your genetic risks.

The medical profession has known for some time that a family history of certain diseases increases the risk of developing them. But as researchers have learned more about human genes, they've found thousands that increase susceptibility to common diseases. The risk of disease increases when these "susceptibility genes" interact with other factors, including exposure to chemicals, illness, behavior, and nutrition. So although your genetic background is not the only factor that determines whether you will develop certain diseases, it plays a major role.

Compile a family medical history. Use the information you gather to help determine whether any diseases appear to run in your family and for which you can take steps to prevent or detect and treat early. Make sure to take all the information you've gathered into account. If several of your relatives died of lung cancer, for example, it could mean that your family is susceptible to lung cancer. But if all were smokers and you are not, you may not be at as great a risk.

Common Life-Threatening Illnesses With a Hereditary Component

Cancers:	Brain	Lung
	Breast	Ovarian
	Colorectal	Prostate
	Endometrial	Skin
	Kidney	Stomach
Cardiovascular diseases:	Atherosclerosis	Hypertension
	Heart disease	Stroke
Diabetes		
Hemochromatosis		
Kidney disease		
Osteoporosis		

Consider carefully genetic testing.

As researchers continue to map the estimated 100,000 human genes, they have learned that as many as 4,000 diseases have a genetic, or inherited, component. In some, such as cystic fibrosis and sickle-cell anemia, genes are directly responsible for the disease. In others, such as breast, colorectal, and ovarian cancers, genes impart a susceptibility to develop the disease.

Along with genes identified as links to diseases, the number of genetic tests available to determine whether a person will develop a certain disease or whether a person is at increased risk is growing. These tests can be both a blessing and a curse.

On the bright side, genetic testing may help further understanding of and, ultimately, treatments for a variety of illnesses. A negative result may take a load off your mind and save you or a family member from needless screening tests (although the lack of a genetic flaw does not necessarily mean that you are immune to a disease). A positive result may give you an opportunity to take steps to reduce your risk of developing a disease, if possible, or to prepare for the possibility that you will develop it.

On the negative side, although genetic tests can accurately detect genetic flaws, they may not be able to tell you whether, or when, those flaws will actually lead to disease. So a positive test result does not tell you the whole story. Likewise, because many diseases have multiple causes, a negative test result does not necessarily preclude disease development. In addition, people who test positively for a genetic flaw may worry about developing the disease or become upset or depressed. And some employers and insurers discriminate against people who are genetically at risk for various diseases.

If you believe you may be at risk for a genetically inherited disease and would like to know what your risk is, check with your doctor to see if a test is available. But before you undergo such a test, make sure you know exactly what the test can and cannot tell you. Make sure you have weighed the pros and cons. And make sure that qualified genetic counseling will be available to you.

Assess your lifestyle and environmental risks.

If you've been blessed with good genes, your lifestyle and environment may be the ultimate determinants of your health. If you've inherited a gene that increases your susceptibility to a certain disease, your lifestyle and environment may increase or decrease your risk of ultimately developing that disease.

The number of such factors that may figure in to your health and longevity is infinite, but you can significantly reduce your risk of a number of life-threatening illnesses by following these three important recommendations.

✔ **Don't smoke.** The single most preventable risk factor for heart disease and stroke is tobacco usage. Although no one knows for sure exactly how tobacco smoke causes heart disease or increases the risk of stroke, smoking has been shown to raise blood pressure and contribute to the development of atherosclerosis. People who smoke have a risk of heart disease two to four times higher than people who don't. Smoking also increases stroke risk by 40 percent in men and 60 percent in women. The good news is that quitting can rapidly reduce your risk of heart disease and stroke. Three years after you quit, your risk of heart disease is almost the same as that of a nonsmoker. Stroke risk declines to that of a nonsmoker within two to five years.

Smoking is also responsible for most lung cancers, and tobacco use contributes to oral, throat, and esophageal cancers. Smoking is also the leading cause of COPD. In fact, 82 percent of those who die of COPD are smokers.

Smoking is also linked to an increased risk of dementia, asthma, hearing loss, and macular degeneration (a leading cause of blindness). All told, smoking contributes to approximately 500,000 deaths a year, according to the Centers for Disease Control and Prevention.

✔ **Maintain a healthy weight.** As many as 97 million Americans are considered overweight. Excess weight—especially around the abdomen—is associated with an increased risk of heart disease. But losing as little as 10 pounds can make a difference. Studies show that in overweight people with high blood pressure, losing weight enhances

the blood pressure-lowering effect of medications, reduces high cholesterol levels, and reduces the need for medications.

Gaining weight as you age may also increase your risk of cancer.
A study that monitored the health of 95,000 nurses for 16 years found
that those who gained weight since age 16 had a higher likelihood of
developing breast cancer. Most at risk were postmenopausal women
who gained 44 to 55 pounds–their risk was increased by as much as a
40 percent.

Being overweight is also associated with an increased risk of diabetes. Up to 90 percent of those with type 2 diabetes are overweight.

✔ *Be physically active.* Exercise strengthens the heart and lowers
heart rate and blood pressure. The American Heart Association (AHA)
suggests a minimum of 30 to 60 minutes of moderate-intensity aerobic activity three to four times a week, augmented with an increase in
lifestyle activities such as taking a walk during your break or using the
stairs. Researchers at Brigham and Women's Hospital in Boston found
that men who exercised 11 to 24 minutes twice a week reduced their
risk of heart attack by 36 percent. Those who did five workouts weekly
reduced their risk by 46 percent. And researchers from the Harvard
School of Public Health recently reported that an hour of moderate
exercise five days a week may lower the risk of stroke by 46 percent.

Exercise is also linked to a reduced risk of cancer and diabetes.
In fact, some researchers have blamed the upsurge in diabetes cases
on Americans' lack of exercise. Thirty minutes of cumulative exercise
daily helps maintain proper glucose levels in the blood. Aerobic exercises such as walking, swimming, and bike riding appear to be most
effective at controlling glucose levels.

 Save your heart, save your life.

According to the National Center for Health Statistics, if all forms of
major cardiovascular diseases were eliminated, life expectancy would
rise by almost 10 years. Unfortunately, experts have not yet found a
way to eliminate heart disease or stroke. They have, however, identified many of the factors that contribute to these diseases. And many
of these risk factors–smoking, high blood pressure, obesity, a sedentary lifestyle, and poor nutrition, for example–can be controlled.

In addition to following the advice in the previous tip, here's what you can do to stay healthy.

✔ **Control high blood pressure.** Approximately one in four Americans has high blood pressure (hypertension), a major risk factor for heart disease and stroke. About half of those individuals don't know they have it. And nearly three-quarters do not have the condition under control.

When your blood pressure is high, your heart has to work harder. This can cause the heart to eventually enlarge from the effort, weakening its ability to pump (a condition called congestive heart failure). High blood pressure also speeds up atherosclerosis, which increases the risk of heart attack and stroke. The kidneys can also be adversely affected by high blood pressure. And a recent National Institute of Aging study even showed brain shrinkage in elderly persons with long-term hypertension.

Your blood pressure is considered high if the systolic pressure (the upper number in a blood pressure reading) is 140 mm Hg or greater and/or the diastolic pressure (the lower number) is 90 mm Hg or greater. Optimal blood pressure is 120 mm Hg/80 mm Hg or below. See chapter 2 for information on how to lower blood pressure with diet.

✔ **Control your cholesterol.** According the AHA, about half of all Americans have unhealthy cholesterol levels. Although we need this soft, fatlike substance to make hormones and build cells, having too much in our blood—particularly too much low-density lipoprotein (LDL) cholesterol—contributes to atherosclerosis. The excess LDL sticks to artery walls, where it oxidizes and begins to form plaque; this buildup, in turn, contributes to heart disease and stroke. The landmark Framingham Heart Study found that heart attack rates rise 2 percent for each 1 percent increase in blood cholesterol, starting at about 200 mg/dL. And according to the AHA, your likelihood of a heart attack doubles if your total cholesterol approaches 300 mg/dL.

The ideal total cholesterol level, according to the National Cholesterol Education Program, is 140 to 200 mg/dL. LDL cholesterol levels should be under 130 mg/dL, and levels of high-density lipoprotein (HDL), which helps escort LDL cholesterol out of the body and lowers heart disease risk, should be above 40 mg/dL. See chapter 2 for ways to reduce your cholesterol levels with diet.

✔ **Get enough antioxidants.** Vitamin E, a potent antioxidant, consistently shows up in studies as a factor in lowering the risk of heart disease. An analysis of studies on the relationship of heart disease and antioxidant consumption, published in the *European Journal of Clinical Nutrition,* showed that those who took in the most antioxidants had a risk of heart disease about 15 percent lower than those who took in the least.

✔ **Reduce blood levels of homocysteine.** Homocysteine, an amino acid believed to damage blood vessels and contribute to fatty plaque buildup in the arteries, is found in high amounts in 40 percent of people with heart disease. It is now considered almost as important a risk factor for heart disease as elevated cholesterol levels. How can you lower your level? Make sure you're getting enough folate and vitamin B_6. Low intake of these vitamins increases blood levels of homocysteine.

✔ **Recognize heart attack symptoms.** Researchers writing in the *British Medical Journal* reported that about two-thirds of people who died of heart attacks didn't recognize the symptoms as such and didn't get help in time. Warning signs include sweating, nausea, pain in the arms and neck, and breathing problems. Few heart attacks actually are preceded by the stereotypical clutching chest pain.

✔ **Consider hormone replacement therapy (HRT).** Estrogen is thought to protect against heart disease by creating beneficial changes in lipids, lipoproteins, and fibrinogen and by triggering favorable vasomotor and antioxidant effects. Numerous studies have confirmed a reduced risk of heart disease in postmenopausal women who used estrogen—one meta-analysis of 17 studies found a 50 percent reduced risk. On a less enthusiastic note, the Heart and Estrogen/Progestin Replacement Study found that the use of HRT by postmenopausal women who already had heart disease did not prevent further heart attacks or death.

 Protect yourself from deadly cancers.

Although the National Cancer Institute estimates that 1.2 million new cases of cancer were diagnosed in 1998, for the first time in history, the rate of breast cancer is down. Lung cancer rates are also decreasing. That's because we now know there are valid ways to avoid cancer, slow its progress, or even cure it. Here are the deadliest cancers and what we know about avoiding them.

Lung cancer. Lung cancer is the leading cause of cancer death among Americans; however, deaths from lung cancer are on the decline. To avoid lung cancer, do not smoke. More than 80 percent of lung cancers are related to smoking. If you live with someone who smokes, you are at risk from secondhand smoke, so help that person stop smoking.

Colorectal cancer. Colorectal cancer is the second leading cause of cancer death among Americans. But colorectal cancer is highly curable if it's caught early. High-fat diets, low rates of activity, and genetics are associated with an increased risk of these cancers. The typical Western-style diet, which is high in red and processed meats and refined sugars and grains and low in fresh fruits and vegetables, doubles the risk of colon cancer, according to a report in the *American Journal of Epidemiology.*

Breast cancer. Breast cancer is second only to lung cancer in cancer deaths among women. But 85 percent of all breast cancer patients—95 percent of those with localized cancer—remain alive five years after the cancer is detected. A woman's risk of breast cancer is related to factors that affect the levels of hormones circulating in her body: age at first menstruation and menopause, number of pregnancies, breast-feeding, obesity, and physical activity. Genetics also play a role.

Prostate cancer. Prostate cancer is the second leading cause of cancer death among American men. The cancer is most common in men over age 70. Appropriate therapy for most forms of slow-growing prostate cancer is still under investigation. Scientists know that prostate cancer is related to male hormones but are uncertain about the exact mechanism that causes the cancer. Since an increase in prostate cancer is associated with animal fats, red meats, and dairy products, saturated fat may be involved.

To reduce your risk of developing these cancers, don't smoke, try to maintain a healthy weight, and get adequate exercise. In addition, heed the following advice.

✔ **Eat a healthy diet.** Eat a low-fat, high-fiber diet that is rich in fruits and vegetables. Studies consistently link a diet high in fruits and vegetables to a lower risk of cancer.

✔ **Get screened.** Regular screening for cancers of the breast, colon, and prostate can reduce mortality. Screening recommendations appear on page 13.

✔ **Consider genetic testing.** If breast, colorectal, or prostate cancer runs in your family, you may wish to consider genetic testing.

✔ **Moderate your alcohol consumption.** Compared with teetotalers, women who regularly have one drink a day raise their breast cancer risk by 11 percent. Those who regularly have more than two raise their risk by 40 percent. Alcohol also contributes to oral and esophageal cancers.

✔ **Consider postmenopausal use of estrogen.** When data gathered from 59,002 postmenopausal participants in the Nurses' Health Study were analyzed, it was found that the risk of colorectal cancer was lower among women receiving hormone replacement therapy. But some studies indicate that HRT may increase the risk of breast cancer.

✔ **Consider the benefits of drug therapy.** Women at high risk of developing breast cancer may wish to consider taking tamoxifen. A recent study of 13,000 high-risk women found that those who used the drug, which is used to treat breast cancer, had a 45 percent reduced incidence of breast cancer. Tamoxifen did raise the risk of endometrial cancer, however. Another drug, raloxifene (Evista), which is used to reduce bone loss, has also shown protective benefits. When 7,705 women were studied, those taking raloxifene had a rate of breast cancer 66 percent lower than those taking a placebo (an inactive substance). They also had a 50 percent lower risk of endometrial cancer.

 Take steps to protect yourself from chronic obstructive pulmonary disease.

Both the incidence of and the number of deaths from COPD are increasing. An estimated 16 million Americans suffered from COPD in 1995, and mortality with severe COPD may be as high as 60 percent at five years. Refrain from smoking and follow the American Lung Association's recommendations to prevent and treat COPD.

✔ *Treat pulmonary infections.*

✔ *Avoid sources of lung irritation.* If the work environment contains large amounts of dust, fumes, and polluted air, it may be necessary to change jobs. Also, check weather reports for information about air quality and amounts of air pollution and restrict activity to early morning or evening on days when the ozone level is high. You may need to stay indoors when pollution levels are dangerous. If you have emphysema, take precautions in cold weather to warm the air that enters your already narrowed lung passages.

✔ *Give your lungs a regular workout.* A therapist can help with breathing exercises to strengthen the muscles used in breathing as part of a pulmonary rehabilitation program.

✔ *Get vaccinated against influenza and pneumococcal pneumonia.* And whenever possible, avoid exposure to colds and influenza at home or in public.

✔ *Get tested for genetic deficiencies.* If you have several family members with emphysema, you may want to have genetic testing performed. An estimated 50,000 to 100,000 Americans with emphysema have a rare inherited form of the disease called alpha 1-antitrypsin (AAT) deficiency-related emphysema. This form of disease is caused by an inherited lack of the lung-protective protein alpha 1-antitrypsin. If you have an AAT deficiency, check with your doctor about AAT replacement therapy.

 Control diabetes risk.

Diabetes is on the upswing in the United States. Between 1980 and 1994, the incidence of new cases increased by 39 percent. In 1998, about 798,000 people were diagnosed with the disease, bringing the total number of Americans who have the disease to 16 million. Yet at least one-third of those with diabetes don't know they have it. Diabetes increases the risk of blindness and limb amputation, as well as kidney and heart disease and stroke.

To avoid the risk of dying early as a result of diabetes, maintain a healthy weight, exercise, and take these additional steps to prevent diabetes or control the risk of complications.

✔ **Get a blood glucose test.** The American Diabetes Association (ADA) calls for routine screening of all Americans starting at age 45 to detect type 2 diabetes. See chart on page 13 for complete screening recommendations.

✔ **Consider estrogen replacement therapy.** New studies have shown that postmenopausal women who take estrogen are less likely to develop diabetes, and if they do, their risk of complications is decreased. A survey of 14,000 postmenopausal women with diabetes showed that those who took the hormone had better blood sugar control, the Kaiser Permanente HMO reported. And a Milwaukee study showed that postmenopausal woman who don't take estrogen are five times more likely to get diabetes than those who do.

If you already have diabetes, you can take the following steps to reduce your risk of life-threatening complications.

✔ **Lower glucose levels.** The United Kingdom Prospective Diabetes Study, the longest and largest study of people with type 2 diabetes, showed that intensive control of blood glucose in type 2 diabetes reduces by 25 percent the chances of developing eye damage potentially leading to blindness and kidney damage leading to kidney failure.

✔ **Control blood pressure.** The U.K. Prospective Diabetes Study also found that aggressive control of high blood pressure in people with type 2 diabetes significantly reduces the risk of heart failure (by 56 percent), stroke (by 44 percent), and death from diabetes (by 32 percent).

✔ **Find coronary artery disease early.** Atherosclerotic damage to the coronary arteries is two to four times more common in people with type 1 diabetes than in the general population. People with diabetes should have their cholesterol levels checked every three to six months. The ADA recommends that people with diabetes keep their cholesterol levels under 200 mg/dL.

✔ **Get immunized.** People with diabetes are more likely to die of complications of influenza such as pneumonia. Deaths among people with diabetes increase 5 to 15 percent during flu epidemics.

SCREENING RECOMMENDATIONS

One of the best ways to prevent an early death is to be screened for diseases that can be prevented or treated early.

The following are general guidelines for medical testing and screening based on various sources, including groups of medical experts and the U.S. Preventive Services Task Force. Keep in mind that there is no agreement among the medical community on what tests should be performed, how often, or if at all. And your own health and family history may suggest a different timetable. You and your doctor should discuss what's best for you.

Cardiovascular Diseases

Blood pressure check: Periodic blood pressure screening is recommended for all people ages 21 and older. Some experts recommend a check every time you visit your doctor.

Cholesterol test: Periodic cholesterol screening is recommended by most groups for men between the ages of 35 and 65 and for women between the ages of 45 and 65. The National Cholesterol Education Program Adult Treatment Panel II recommends testing at least once every five years for all adults ages 20 and older.

Electrocardiogram (EKG): Some experts recommend getting a baseline EKG at age 40 to use as a comparison with future EKGs.

Cancers

Breast cancer: The Task Force recommends screening every one to two years with mammography alone or mammography and an annual clinical breast exam for women ages 50 to 69. Most other groups now recommend that mammograms be given every one to two years beginning at age 40 and every year beginning at age 50. Also recommended are an annual clinical breast exam and monthly breast self-exams.

(continued on next page)

(continued)

Cervical cancer: A Pap test at least once every three years is the recommendation for women who are sexually active or who are 18 years or older. The American Cancer Society, National Cancer Institute, American College of Obstetricians and Gynecologists, and American Academy of Family Physicians recommend annual tests but permit testing less frequently at the discretion of a physician after three or more annual tests have been normal.

Colorectal cancer: Virtually every group recommends regular screening for all people ages 50 and older. The American Cancer Society recommends an annual digital rectal exam beginning at age 40, an annual fecal occult blood test beginning at age 50, and sigmoidoscopy every three to five years beginning at age 50.

Prostate cancer: The American Cancer Society and the American Urological Association recommend an annual digital rectal exam beginning at age 40 and an annual prostate-specific antigen (PSA) blood test beginning at age 50. The digital rectal exam is limited in detecting cancer, however. And experts have not reached a consensus on the use of the PSA test (which measures levels of PSA in the blood) in accurately diagnosing cancer. The test fails to detect 20 percent of prostate cancers and cannot distinguish among prostate cancer and more benign prostate conditions.

Skin cancer: The American Cancer Society recommends monthly skin self-examinations for all adults and physician-administered skin examination every three years for people ages 20 to 39 and annually for people ages 40 and older.

Diabetes

Blood glucose test: The American Diabetes Association recommends a blood glucose test for people who are obese, have a family history of diabetes, are of African-American, Hispanic, or Native American ancestry, have high blood pressure, have delivered a baby weighing more than nine pounds, or had gestational diabetes.

Keep your immunizations up-to-date.

Each year, 50,000 to 70,000 adults die of diseases that are preventable with vaccinations. According to a report given at the American College of Physicians' 1998 annual meeting, some 34,000 lives could be saved if all adults were immunized. Experts say vaccines can prevent 70 percent of influenza deaths, 60 percent of cases of a certain type of pneumonia, and 90 percent of cases of hepatitis B.

But at least half of all Americans are behind on their booster shots, and new vaccines that prevent death from influenza, pneumonia, and hepatitis B are often underutilized.

Here are the Centers for Disease Control and Prevention's recommended immunizations for adults.

Chicken pox (Varicella): Two doses, four to eight weeks apart, are recommended for people ages 13 and older who have not had chicken pox. This common childhood disease does occur in adults, and serious complications are possible.

Hepatitis A: Two doses, six to 12 months apart, are recommended for those traveling abroad and those at risk (health care workers, partners and close contacts of people with hepatitis A, IV drug users, and hemodialysis patients).

Hepatitis B: Three doses, the second a month after the first and the third five months after the second, are recommended for those at risk (health care workers, partners and close contacts of people with hepatitis B, IV drug users, and hemodialysis patients).

Influenza: A yearly injection in the fall is recommended for people ages 65 and older, for people with chronic conditions such as heart disease, lung disease, kidney disease, and diabetes, and for people who live with at-risk individuals. The risk of dying from flu-associated complications rises as you get older, but the CDC estimates that 80 percent of deaths from such complications in the elderly can be prevented by immunization.

Measles, Mumps, Rubella (MMR): Two doses, one month apart, are recommended for adults born after 1956 if immunity cannot be proved. Although they are considered childhood diseases, they also occur in adults.

Pneumococcal pneumonia: One dose is recommended for people ages 65 and older and for people with chronic conditions, kidney disorders, or sickle-cell anemia. Pneumonococcal infections kill 40,000 people annually through sepsis (infection of blood or tissues) and meningitis and are becoming increasingly resistant to antibiotics.

Tetanus/Diphtheria: Three doses plus a booster every 10 years are recommended for all adults if the initial series was not given in childhood. If you have a contaminated wound, especially from rusty metal or gardening, your doctor may recommend a tetanus shot if your last booster was five or more years ago. Children typically receive a combined diphtheria, tetanus, and pertussis vaccine, yet about half of all adults over age 60 never received the diphtheria immunization or periodic booster shots.

The Savvy Health Care Consumer

 Know your rights.

By knowing your medical rights, you can help avoid many of the errors, mistakes, and risks too often associated with medical care. Studies show that close to 10 percent of all consumers admitted to hospitals acquire an infection they did not have before admission, and up to 80,000 people die each year as a result. It's estimated that nearly 90,000 people die each year as a result of hospital negligence. And close to 40 percent of all people in American hospitals are there as a result of something a doctor did to them. According to some experts, health care is the fourth leading cause of death in the United States, not far behind heart disease, cancer, and stroke.

No matter what the medical setting, you have the right to say "no" to a test, treatment, or procedure; discharge yourself from a hospital even if your doctor or other hospital personnel think it's wrong; and change your doctor or get a second opinion in a hospital, even if you're in the middle of treatment. If you're not satisfied with a health maintenance organization's (HMO's) decision regarding care, you have the right to appeal. And if your insurance company denies a claim, you can challenge that decision not just within the plan itself, but with your state insurance department.

While we certainly do not have the room to list all your medical rights in this book, we do think you should be aware of some important issues related to your rights, starting with the most fundamental one of all.

Informed consent. Before undergoing any medical test, surgical procedure, or other treatment, you are entitled to be informed about it in detail. Your health care provider must explain – preferably in writing – the following:

- What your condition is
- The test, procedure, or treatment being recommended
- Exactly what is involved in the test, procedure, or treatment
- The expected benefits of the treatment
- The risks of the treatment
- How likely the treatment is to succeed
- Alternative treatment options (and the risks associated with them), including the option of no treatment at all

Advocates to work on your behalf. It's very difficult to exercise your medical rights if you're sick. Usually a family member or a trusted friend, your advocate will intervene with your health care providers when something is wrong or will ask the questions you are unable (or afraid) to ask. It is your legal right to have a family member or friend (anyone you designate) with you in the doctor's examining room and at your bedside in the hospital 24 hours a day. The only restriction is that your advocate cannot interfere with a medical professional's ability to deliver medical care.

If you need further help while in the hospital, find out if the facility has a patient representative. This person helps patients with difficult problems that haven't been solved through the usual channels. Patient representatives intervene with hospital management to get problems resolved.

Your health care provider as advocate. You have the right to expect your physician or other health professional to be your advocate when dealing with health insurance claim denials or other disputes you may be having within the system. If you're having trouble getting an appointment with a specialist, ask (and expect) your primary care doctor to intervene. See the appendix for a list of resources that provide information about health care rights.

 ## Keep watch over your medical records.

Your medical record is an important component of your lifetime of medical treatment. One inaccuracy—not listing an allergy to a particular medication, for example—could prove fatal. Therefore, another key to a long, healthy life is making sure you know what's in your record and that the information is accurate.

Information in your medical records belongs to you, although the original records stay with the provider. You are entitled to look at your records and have them explained to you at any time. Twenty-six states have actual laws that allow you access to copies of your records. But even in states that do not have laws, medical providers must allow you to see your record and to have copies of it. (Of course, there may be a copying charge.)

If your doctor, hospital, or other medical entity refuses to give you a copy of your record, file a complaint with your state attorney general's office.

To make sure the medical information in your record is accurate, follow these tips.

✔ *Get copies of your records from your health care providers.* Check them carefully to assure they are accurate. If they aren't, talk to the doctor or facility who created the record and have him justify any entry you question.

If you have ever applied for life insurance and taken a physical exam, it's likely that information about your health is stored with the Medical Information Bureau (MIB), a repository of information for the insurance industry. Wrong information in this file could mean being turned down for future coverage. Call the MIB at 617-426-3660 to find out how to get the information in your files and how to correct any inaccuracies.

📬 **Track your own medical history.** In today's world, where you might see scores of doctors over a lifetime, be admitted to numerous hospitals or outpatient facilities, and use many medications, keeping your own medical record is a great way to make sure all the important information is one place. Use your record, too, to double-check the records kept by others.

 Educate yourself.

The more you know about your medical conditions and health in general, the better your chances to live to 100. Studies show that consumers who are knowledgeable about their conditions, the care they're receiving, and the options available to them get better medical results.

Here's what to do to keep on top of the trends and developments that can affect your health.

📬 **Use the Internet.** No time to go to a medical library? Hundreds of thousands of consumers use the government's National Library of Medicine search service to access the 9 million citations in the periodicals database called MEDLINE. The Web page address is www.ncbi.nlm.nih.gov/PubMed/.

While on the Web, check out chat groups focusing on the condition or issue that interests you. For example, women who have had breast cancer maintain several chat groups where they share information, answer each other's questions, and refer people to other sites and resources.

📬 **Get a book.** Books can't keep current on weekly advances in medicine, but they are good foundations for basic health information. Look for ones published by major medical institutions such as Columbia University or the Mayo Clinic. *The Merck Manual of Medical Information—Home Edition** is a top-rated consumer guide to major health conditions. You can also rely on the more than 80 books written or published by the People's Medical Society. These books range

---

* Whitehouse Station, N.J.: Merck Research Laboratories, 1997.

from titles such as *Take This Book to the Hospital With You** (an in-depth consumer guide to surviving a hospital stay) to *Prostate: Questions You Have . . . Answers You Need*.†

✔ **Use your pharmacy as a resource.** By law, pharmacists are now required to privately counsel you about your prescription if you request it. They should also provide printed information about each prescription.

✔ **Call reputable organizations.** Federal and state organizations such as the Centers for Disease Control and Prevention and state health departments, some physician trade organizations, and organizations such as the American Cancer Society and the American Diabetes Association provide consumer-oriented resource materials.

✔ **Understand medical studies.** Medical researchers are constantly finding new and exciting ways to improve human health, but each completed study is only a part of the picture and rarely has a final, definitive answer to complex medical questions. Rather than relying on news reports of health studies, if you're really interested in a subject or condition, look at the study itself. How can you get the most from such a reading? Study the brief summary of findings generally published at the beginning of a study. Then go directly to the end of the study to the section often labeled "conclusion" or "discussion of findings." Once you've concluded your research—including perhaps taking a look at some of the references listed at the end of the study—take the information you've found to the doctors or caregivers who are treating you. Hopefully, this will initiate a productive and educational conversation with them.

A word to the wise: Make sure you know the validity of the source of the study and the journal or publication in which it appears. Obviously, studies from well-known universities or in publications such as the *Journal of the American Medical Association* or the *New England Journal of Medicine* are among the most reputable.

---

* Allentown, Pa.: People's Medical Society, 1997.
† Allentown, Pa.: People's Medical Society, 1996.

Choose the right doctor.

A competent, skilled doctor is critical for the proper treatment of medical conditions that inevitably happen to everyone. In a People's Medical Society survey of people who reached the age of 100, we discovered that most, at some time or another, had suffered from major medical conditions such as cancer and heart disease. Each of them felt that having competent doctors working as their partners was instrumental in reaching the century mark.

Here are some key things to remember when you're selecting a doctor–be it a primary care physician or a specialist.

✔ **Choose the right doc for the right condition.** Choosing a specialist rather than a generalist can work to your benefit or detriment. If you have a specific problem or a chronic condition such as asthma or diabetes, you can work with a doctor who spends the majority of her time dealing with those problems. But many specialists know very little about conditions other than those in their area of expertise and might not give you the best care for other conditions. So make sure you use the doctor that's most appropriate for your condition. That includes a good primary care physician as well as specialists as your condition warrants.

✔ **Know qualifications.**

■ Where did the doctor go to medical school? This includes internship and residency–the training after medical school. A medical degree from Harvard or Johns Hopkins is nice, but many fine physicians have graduated from less famous medical schools. On the other hand, top schools often produce top clinicians–ones who are on the cutting edge of medical practice.

■ Is the physician board certified? Most medical specialties have organizations that certify doctors in that specialty. These specialty boards establish a list of criteria the individual must meet in order to gain certification. This usually involves postgraduate education, ongoing continuing education, and other peer review processes. While board certification does not assure or guarantee competence or high quality, it does show that the doctor is interested in his field, continues to keep abreast of current trends, and is willing to be reviewed. To find out if your doctor is board certified, contact the American Board of Medical Specialties at 800-776-CERT.

■ What's the doctor's experience? While a hotshot new doctor right out of a fancy medical residency may have the latest information and the most energy, experience in medicine goes a long way. A study reported in the journal *Circulation* showed that balloon angioplasty, a technique for clearing blocked arteries, is safest in experienced hands. Doctors who performed fewer than 70 angioplasties annually had a complication rate three times that of doctors who did the procedure at least 270 times annually. The study suggested that patients can reduce the risk of complications—which can be life-threatening—by 69 percent if they choose more experienced physicians.

✔ *Check out a doctor's reputation.* Many unsuspecting consumers have been treated—and harmed—by doctors of poor repute.

■ Call your state medical licensing board. Find out if the board (usually located in your state capital) has taken any action against the doctor or has any action pending. If you know that the doctor has practiced in another state, call the board in that state as well.

■ Check the courts. Medical malpractice lawsuits are filed in local courts, so check the court records in the communities (usually counties) where the doctor practices. If any lawsuits have been brought against the doctor, see how they've been resolved. If they were settled, ask the doctor to explain the situation and what happened.

■ Ask other doctors. Asking another doctor about a colleague can be helpful. Doctors know a great deal about other doctors in town, but most are reluctant to give you a candid appraisal of their work. The question to ask is, "Have you or a member of your family ever been treated by Dr. X, and would you use him again?"

■ Ask a nurse. Nurses are wonderful sources of information about doctors. Nurses often know the behind-the-scenes story and can give insider tips. We recommend asking nurses about specific doctors. A good place to start is the question, "Would you use this doctor yourself for my condition?"

Choose safe hospitals.

It's been said that a hospital is the worst place to be when you're sick. The risks to life associated with a hospital stay are many. Nearly 90,000 people a year die as a result of hospital negligence. And up to 80,000 die of hospital-acquired infections. Therefore, it is essential that you choose the safest and most appropriate hospital for your needs.

✔ **Find out how often the hospital treats your condition.** As with doctors, the more often hospitals deal with a condition or perform a procedure within their walls, the better the chances they'll get it right the first time. The more experienced hospital personnel become, the better they are able to deal with complications or problems that might arise.

✔ **Find out about accreditation.** Most hospitals are accredited by the Joint Commission on Accreditation of Healthcare Organizations (JCAHO), but some only after many corrections to problems discovered. Quality Check, a new service offered by the JCAHO, provides you with the JCAHO's findings on individual hospitals, surgery centers, and nursing homes, but not all inspected or accredited facilities participate. To learn more, contact the JCAHO at 1 Renaissance Blvd., Oakbrook Terrace, IL 60181; 630-792-5000 or visit its Web site at www.jcaho.org/qualitycheck/.

✔ **Tour your local hospitals.** Do this when you're healthy and not in need of care. Does the equipment seem state-of-the-art? Is the place clean? Do patient room areas smell of urine or worse? Are hospital personnel caring for patients or hanging around the halls doing nothing? If you see any patients, ask them how they'd rate their care. Are nurses responding promptly to their calls? Are procedures and other matters explained? Are the patients kept up all night by hall noise?

✔ **Ask questions of the hospital administrator and/or the physician who serves as medical director.** Ask what the hospital's infection rate is. Find out the hospital's mortality (death) rate by procedure or for the specific procedure you might undergo. Ask about the morbidity (complication) rate by procedure. In other words, get as much information about the quality and outcomes of their care as possible. Good hospitals save lives and extend your life span. And obviously, you want to be at the best hospital you can find. That may mean you should look beyond your local area. Institutions such as the Cleveland Clinic, Memorial Sloan-Kettering Cancer Center in New York City, and the Mayo Clinic in Rochester, Minnesota, have international reputations for the diagnosis and treatment of specific illnesses and conditions. In some cases, it may be worth your while to use such facilities. One of the best ways to learn about these well-known facilities is by using *U.S. News and World Report*'s annual ranking of what it terms the "best hospitals in America." By collecting data from a variety of sources, the magazine lists the best hospitals overall—and the best in various specialties, including cancer, cardiology, endocrinology, gastroenterology, gynecology, neurology, pulmonary disease, and urology.

In addition, the American Hospital Directory provides on-line, comparative data for most hospitals from Medicare claims data, cost reports, and other public use files from the federal Health Care Financing Administration. For more information, contact the American Hospital Directory, 620 W. Main St., Suite 200A, Louisville, KY 40202; 800-577-8070 or visit its Web site at www.ahd.com/guest1.html.

 Know your health plan.

Do you have a deductible? Will you be reimbursed for out-of-network care? What's the copayment for emergency room visits? What is preauthorization, and how do you obtain it? If you receive health coverage from your employer, your company's personnel office should have materials that explain all aspects of your coverage. Your insurer's member services department can also answer these and all other questions related to your plan.

If you are a Medicare or Medicaid beneficiary, be sure to get the informative brochures put out by the Health Care Financing Administration (the federal agency that administers those programs). Those brochures are available at all Social Security offices, as well as at most senior citizen centers, county Area Agency on Aging offices, and local welfare offices.

Be well insured.

Research has found that being insured is an important factor in staying healthy. A study published in the *Journal of the American Medical Association*, for example, compared mortality rates of people who were privately insured with those of people who had no insurance. At the end of the 12-year follow-up period, 9.6 percent of the insured people had died and 18.4 percent of the uninsured had died. In short, that lack of insurance doubled the rate of mortality. A study published in the *Annals of Internal Medicine* showed that people with employer-provided health insurance had mortality rates 20 to 30 percent lower than working people without insurance.

But not all insurance plans are created equal, a report in the *Journal of the American College of Cardiology* concluded. The type of health insurance, for example, appears to play a role in the treatment heart attack patients receive. A study of people older than 65 who had suffered heart attacks found that those with traditional fee-for-service insurance plans were about two times more likely to undergo angiography, a diagnostic x-ray used to identify clogged coronary arteries, than were patients who were on Medicaid or those who had no insurance. Fee-for-service patients also were 30 percent more likely to have diagnostic angiograms and other cardiac procedures such as bypass surgery or angioplasty to open clogged arteries than patients in HMOs. Researchers also pointed out that hospitalized fee-for-service patients were 55 percent less likely to die than Medicaid patients.

Your type of insurance plan also influences your odds of having access to the medications that may help keep you alive, especially if you are older. In one study, elderly people were up to 17 percent more likely to be getting prescription drug treatment if they had private insurance that covered such costs.

The bottom line: Buy the most health insurance you can afford, but do not duplicate your coverage.

Here's what to look for when considering a health insurance policy or managed care plan.

Services. What's covered and what's not? Does the plan have any special programs for chronic illnesses? Will it provide the medical equipment and medications you need? What does it exclude? And what about experimental procedures or medications?

Who's included. If you're considering a fee-for-service plan, make sure your doctor will accept the insurance company's reimbursement as payment in full (less any required copayments or deductibles). If you're considering a managed care plan such as an HMO, find out if your current providers are in the plan—the same with your favorite hospitals or a particular medical specialist.

Who pays. Are there deductibles? What do you pay after the deductible is met? What are the copayments? If you are in a managed care plan, will the plan pay if you go out of its physician or hospital network? How much is paid for services received from out-of-network providers? Is there a lifetime cap or annual limit on what will be paid? Do you have to get preapproval before major procedures are covered? Do you have to get preauthorization to use an emergency room or an out-of-state doctor or facility if you're out of town?

Quality judgments. The National Committee for Quality Assurance (NCQA) accredits HMOs and other managed care organizations. Three-fourths of the HMO plans that Americans are enrolled in have been reviewed by the NCQA. To learn about your plan, call 888-275-7585 for an accreditation status list or check out the NCQA Web site at www.info.ncqa.org/status.htm.

Prescription drug coverage. Close to 85 percent of all physician visits end with a prescription being written. So if you can buy it and afford it, purchase prescription drug insurance or opt for it through your employer. It may make a difference both in your ability to get well and your ability to live longer.

 Use medications wisely.

Every year, thousands of deaths occur when consumers have adverse reactions to the very medications designed to help them. Many of these fatalities can be avoided if drugs are prescribed and used correctly. Here's how to use life-saving medications wisely.

✔ *Fill your prescriptions.* About half of all prescriptions are never filled. Maybe the medication is too expensive, you're feeling better already, or you experienced side effects the last time you took the drug. Whatever the reason, talk to your doctor before you decide not to fill a prescription. Perhaps she can find a less expensive drug for the problem. Let your doctor know immediately if side effects occur. She can cut down on the dosage, switch you to another medication, or offer some other alternative.

✔ *Beware of similar drug names.* Almost 20,000 drugs are available in the United States, and at least 600 of them have similar names. For example, the drug Feldene treats arthritis, while Seldane treats allergies. And Zantac treats ulcers, while Xanax relieves anxiety. Be sure you know what prescription your doctor ordered and whether it is appropriate for your condition.

✔ *Double-check your prescriptions.* Each day in the United States, 46,000 prescription errors are made in retail pharmacies. Similar packaging and labeling account for almost half of the errors reported to the U.S. Pharmacopeia, a nonprofit organization that sets drug standards and collects information about prescribing errors. Make sure the prescription you pick up at the pharmacy is exactly what your doctor ordered. Confirm verbally with the pharmacist the name of the product, the dosage, and the number of pills or amount of liquid dispensed. Check that against what your doctor wrote down. That means you should always ask your doctor to write down, in plain English, exactly what he is ordering from the pharmacy.

✔ *Communicate with your health care provider.* Let your doctor or other health care provider know what medications you are taking, including over-the-counter remedies and vitamin supplements. You want to make sure that the mix of products does not produce a serious or fatal reaction. And ask your doctor for details about the medication he prescribed, possible side effects, what to do if you miss a dose, warnings, and interactions. Ask the same questions of your pharmacist.

✔ *Follow instructions carefully.* Some pharmacy experts suggest that half of all medications are used improperly. Unless you are experiencing a negative reaction or side effect, it's not wise to stop taking a prescription medication just because the symptoms go away. The cause of the problem may still be present in your body, and the full course of the medication may be needed to completely eliminate the problem. For the medications to work best, try to follow the time periods when a drug should be taken. If you're supposed to take a pill with each meal, it's presumed to mean breakfast, lunch, and dinner—between five and six hours apart.

✔ **Store your medications properly.** The worst place to store medications is the place most people use—the bathroom medicine cabinet. A bathroom's heat and humidity are bad for everything from antibiotics to eyedrops. A secure box stored in a bedroom (away from sunlight and children) is a better choice.

✔ **Look up your medications.** The more you know about the medications you are taking, the better you will understand how the drugs work, what problems may arise, and if there are any specific warnings that apply to you. For some people, owning a so-called pill book might be a good idea. The most comprehensive (and most expensive) is the *Physician's Desk Reference*,* also called the *PDR*. The consumer version of the *PDR* is the *Physician's Desk Reference Family Guide to Prescription Drugs*.† You also can go on-line to the U.S. Pharmacopeia Web site at www.usp.org/toolbar/search.htm#check.

✔ **Use the same pharmacy.** Try to fill all your prescriptions at the same pharmacy or at a chain pharmacy that keeps computer records on all its customers. That way, the pharmacist who is filling your order will be able to see what other medications you are taking and avoid any dangerous conflicts. Most chain stores and many independent pharmacies have computer programs that automatically alert the pharmacist if you are being given a drug that might negatively interact with one you are already taking. However, the store must know what you're taking in order for this to be effective.

✔ **Be vigilant in the hospital.** Pick a family member or friend to keep an eye on what drugs you are receiving. And make sure that the nurse who gives you your medication double-checks your patient I.D. bracelet every time you receive drugs. If you have any drug allergies,

---

* Montvale, N.J.: Medical Economics Co., 1998.
† Montvale, N.J.: Medical Economics Co., 1998.

let the person providing the medication know. It's also a good idea to put a note with the information over your bed.

🗸 *Follow directions for over-the-counter* (OTC) *drugs.* More than 100,000 OTC medications are available, from cold and cough medications to pain relievers. Since these drugs can be obtained without a prescription and are usually not supervised by a health care provider, the Food and Drug Administration permits only the safest ones to be sold. Despite the safety record for OTCs, though, you need to pay attention to dosage, side effects, interactions with other drugs, and when to take the medications. These are all clearly written on the packaging.

 Avoid unnecessary surgery.

Every year, more than 27 million people enter hospitals for medical procedures. Another 31.5 million have outpatient surgery. Out of that 58 million, it has been suggested that almost one-sixth of the operations are unnecessary.

How can you find out if your physician has recommended a surgery that isn't medically useful? Be wary of the most common surgeries: back surgery, cataract surgery, cesarean section, coronary bypass surgery, foot surgery, gallbladder surgery, hip surgery, hysterectomy, knee surgery, prostate surgery, and tonsillectomy. There is great controversy about when such operations are absolutely necessary. And because each procedure carries risks, including the risk of death, it is essential that you get a diagnostic second opinion (one that confirms what's wrong) as well as a treatment second opinion (one that confirms the proposed treatment). Studies show that up to 20 percent of diagnostic second opinions do not confirm first opinions and up to 80 percent (in knee surgery, for example) of treatment second opinions disagree.

2 Nutrition, Hormones, and Supplements

Hippocrates was right in counseling, "Let food be your medicine." Experts believe that 40 percent of cancers in men and 60 percent of cancers in women are related to diet. Researchers are increasingly finding a strong association between increased dietary fat and cancers of the breast, ovary, endometrium, prostate, and colon. A diet high in fat has also been shown to contribute to heart disease and stroke, and insufficient amounts of certain minerals can increase the risk of diseases such as osteoporosis.

But while a poor diet increases the risk of disease—and, consequently, death—a good diet can reduce the risk of disease and add years to your life. Research on vitamins and minerals is pinpointing many of these nutrients that may play roles in preventing and fighting chronic conditions such as heart disease, cancer, and diabetes, as well as deficiency diseases. As a result, the Recommended Dietary Allowances (RDAs), which were designed to prevent deficiencies, are being replaced by recommendations that focus on the role of nutrients in optimizing health. And a very-low-fat diet, combined with a program of exercise and stress management, has actually been found in several studies to *reverse* atherosclerosis.

There is much you can do to add years to your life instead of pounds to your middle.

Healthy Eating Habits

 Follow the "Dietary Guidelines for Americans."

The "Dietary Guidelines for Americans," which are published by the U.S. Department of Agriculture and updated every five years to incorporate the latest advances in medical and scientific research, form the basis for the Food Guide Pyramid, the "Nutrition Facts" panels that appear on nearly every food in your supermarket, and federal nutrition policy and programs.

The current guidelines, published in 1995, are based on the following general recommendations: You should eat a variety of foods; balance the food you eat with physical activity to maintain or improve your weight; eat plenty of grain products, vegetables, and fruits; eat a diet that is low in cholesterol and fat, especially saturated fat; moderate your intake of sugar, salt, and sodium; and drink alcoholic beverages only in moderation.

Specific recommendations appear in the Food Guide Pyramid (shown on opposite page), which was created to help consumers visualize how the guidelines translate into a daily diet.

Food labels can also help simplify your efforts to follow the guidelines. Here are the major components of food labels and tips on how to use them to improve your eating habits.

Serving size. This is the amount upon which the other figures are based. Watch this closely when you are counting calories. For example, the serving size for cereal may be one-half cup, but a large cereal bowl will hold much more than that. Use a measuring cup to ensure that your portions aren't too big or too small.

Percent Daily Value. Percent Daily Value tells you what percentage of your recommended daily allotment (or Daily Value) of certain nutrients are in a food if you eat 2,000 calories per day. This tool can help you compare different foods without performing any calculations. A high percentage means the food contains a lot of a particular nutrient; a low percentage means it contains a little. Depending on the nutrient, your goal should be to choose foods that together give you close to or no more than 100 percent of each nutrient for a day or an

Food Guide Pyramid

A Guide to Daily Food Choices

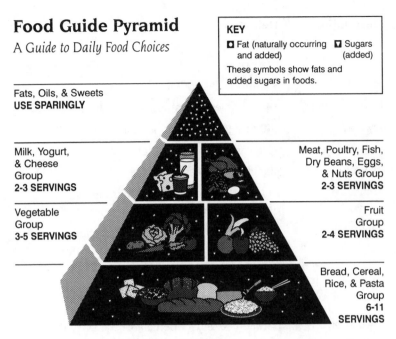

KEY

□ Fat (naturally occurring ▼ Sugars
and added) (added)

These symbols show fats and
added sugars in foods.

Fats, Oils, & Sweets
USE SPARINGLY

Milk, Yogurt,
& Cheese
Group
2-3 SERVINGS

Meat, Poultry, Fish,
Dry Beans, Eggs,
& Nuts Group
2-3 SERVINGS

Vegetable
Group
3-5 SERVINGS

Fruit
Group
2-4 SERVINGS

Bread, Cereal,
Rice, & Pasta
Group
**6-11
SERVINGS**

Source: U.S. Department of Agriculture/U.S. Department of Health and Human Services

Note: A range of servings is given for each food group. The smaller number is for people
who consume about 1,600 calories a day; the larger number is for those who consume
about 2,800 calories a day.

average of about 100 percent a day over a few days. Nutrients for
which Percent Daily Values are provided include total fat, saturated
fat, cholesterol, sodium, total carbohydrate, dietary fiber, sugars, proteins, vitamins A and C, calcium, and iron.

Ingredients listing. Food labels also have to list ingredients—important information for someone who is avoiding certain foods for health,
religious, or other reasons. Chief ingredients are listed first.

In addition to these mandated items, food labels can also include these claims.

Nutrient claims. Foods can be described by their levels of certain
nutrients, including fat, calories, sodium, sugar, vitamins, and minerals. The chart on the following page defines these descriptions as they
apply to a single serving of food.

Description	Definition
free	No amount or a trivial amount of a nutrient or calories
low fat	3 grams or less of fat
low saturated fat	1 gram or less of saturated fat
low sodium	140 milligrams or less of sodium
low cholesterol	20 milligrams or less of saturated fat
low calorie	40 calories or less
reduced	At least 25 percent less of a nutrient or of calories than the regular product
light (lite)	One-third fewer calories or half the fat of the regular product or half the sodium content of a low-fat, low-calorie food
high	20 percent or more of the Daily Value of a particular nutrient
good source	Between 10 and 19 percent of the Daily Value of a particular nutrient
less	25 percent less of a nutrient or of calories than another food

Health claims. These claims, which are strictly regulated by the Food and Drug Administration (FDA), link a nutrient or food to the risk of a chronic disease. Thus far, the only links approved by the FDA are calcium and osteoporosis; fat and cancer; saturated fat and cholesterol and heart disease; fiber and cancer; fiber and heart disease; sodium and high blood pressure; fruits and vegetables and cancer; and folic acid and neural tube defects (a type of birth defect).

 Monitor your fat intake.

Although fat is often the enemy of good health—it promotes obesity and heart disease—some fat is necessary in the diet.

Fat is a storehouse of extra calories in the body. Its balloonlike cells insulate and cushion internal organs, maintain healthy hair and skin, carry the fat-soluble vitamins A, D, E, and K, regulate blood cholesterol, and supply materials for growth and development and hormones such as prostaglandins that control blood pressure. So it's clearly not desirable to eliminate all fat from your diet.

Too much fat—well, you already know from chapter 1 what diseases it's in cahoots with. A high-fat diet also crowds out the nutrients you should be getting from foods such as vegetables and fruit.

Here's a rundown of the various types of fats and how they affect your health.

Saturated fats. Found in foods such as meats, butter, pastries, pizza, gravy, and foods made with lard, these fats stay solid at room temperature. They cause your liver to manufacture excess cholesterol, which raises your total cholesterol level as well as your level of low-density lipoprotein (LDL), the so-called bad cholesterol. High total and LDL cholesterol levels contribute to atherosclerosis. High saturated fat intake also increases risk of colorectal, prostate, endometrial, and, possibly, breast cancers.

Polyunsaturated fats. Liquid or soft at room temperature, these fats include corn and safflower oils and the omega-3 fatty acids found in cold-water fish. Polyunsaturated fats reduce total cholesterol, but they also reduce high-density lipoprotein (HDL), the so-called good cholesterol.

Monounsaturated fats. These fats, which are liquid at room temperature, include heart-healthy oils such as canola, peanut, and olive. Studies have found that olive and canola oils may reduce LDL without reducing HDL.

Trans fats. Because unsaturated fats are typically liquid, the food industry often hydrogenates them to make them harder and help keep them from becoming rancid. Hydrogenation turns unsaturated fats into trans fatty acids, or trans fats, which are found in margarine, fried foods, and baked goods. Research now shows that trans fats are as unhealthy as saturated fats because they lower HDL and raise LDL. Trans fats also increase triglycerides (the chemical form in which fat exists in food and in the body) and increase Lp(a), a protein that contributes to atherosclerosis and blood clots.

Many experts believe that trans fats should be limited. Unfortunately, it's not always easy to detect the presence of trans fats in foods because they are often listed as unsaturated fat. Nutrition interest groups such as the Center for Science in the Public Interest are encouraging the Food and Drug Administration to include trans fats in the saturated fat category on food labels because these fats raise LDL levels. In order to avoid trans fats, look for the term "partially hydro-genated vegetable oil" on food labels. Reduce your consumption of foods that use trans fats for preparation: fried foods, including dough-nuts, chicken, and french fries; and baked goods, including cookies, crackers, and pies. And choose soft rather than solid margarine.

 Lower your cholesterol with diet.

Although some people have inherited disorders that keep their cho-lesterol levels high, most people can reduce their cholesterol with diet. Reducing your intake of fat–particularly saturated fat–can do more to lower cholesterol than reducing your intake of dietary choles-terol itself.

If your cholesterol levels are high, the National Cholesterol Education Program (NCEP) suggests that you follow its Step 1 Diet. With this diet, your total fat intake should be no more than 30 per-cent of your daily calories and your saturated fat intake should be be-tween 8 and 10 percent. Dietary cholesterol intake should be less than 300 milligrams per day, and you should take in just enough cal-ories to maintain your weight. If the Step 1 Diet fails to lower your cholesterol levels, if you have heart disease, or if you are at risk of de-veloping heart disease, the NCEP suggests the Step 2 Diet. This diet retains a total fat intake of no more than 30 percent of calories but re-stricts saturated fat intake to less than 7 percent of total calories and dietary cholesterol intake to less than 200 milligrams per day (that's less than the cholesterol in one large egg).

 Go fishing for adequate amounts of omega-3 oils.

Although Greenland Eskimos eat about a pound of fatty fish and whale meat daily, they have few heart attacks. Other populations who eat a lot of fish also have a reduced rate of death from heart disease. Credit omega-3 oils.

Found in fish that eat aquatic plants, especially those fish that live in cold waters, these polyunsaturated oils lower triglycerides and reduce the tendency of platelets to clump together and stick to artery walls, which increases the likelihood of blood clot formation. (Blood clots increase the risk of heart attack and ischemic stroke.)

Fish oils are also beneficial to those with existing heart disease. According to a study reported in the *Canadian Journal of Physiology and Pharmacology*, people with blocked coronary arteries and irregular heartbeats (arrhythmias) had lower rates of death from heart disease when they made fish oil a regular part of their diet. Fish oil has been shown to reduce ventricular arrhythmias. Other studies have shown that it lowers blood pressure.

How can you increase the omega-3 in your diet? Use fish oil supplements, is the American Heart Association's (AHA's) recommendation to people with high triglyceride levels whose medications are not effective. But others should get their omega-3 fish oils from the fish themselves—salmon, albacore tuna, swordfish, sardines, mackerel, and hard shellfish.

For some people, omega-3 supplements may be risky. Omega-3 blocks a substance in the body that makes blood platelet cells sticky and also inhibits production of platelet activating factor. This may raise the risk of hemorrhagic stroke and increase bleeding during surgery or after trauma. People with bleeding disorders, those taking anticoagulants, and those with uncontrolled hypertension (who already are at risk for stroke) shouldn't take fish oil supplements, the *University of California at Berkeley Wellness Letter* advises. Consuming two helpings of fish weekly, rather than daily fish oil supplements, avoids this possibility, according to the American Dietetic Association.

 ## Lower blood pressure with diet.

What you eat and drink can raise—or lower—your blood pressure. Here are some dietary steps you can take to lower your blood pressure.

✔ **Monitor your sodium intake.** Sodium, the mineral that makes up 40 percent of table salt, acts as an electrolyte—an electrically charged particle that helps regulate blood pressure and volume. Sodium causes your body to hold on to fluids. This makes the blood's volume increase and the heart work harder. If there is too much volume and the blood vessels don't expand enough, high blood pressure is the result. Up to 30 percent of Americans have sodium-sensitive blood pressure, according to the American Dietetic Association. For these people, too much sodium in the diet contributes to high blood pressure.

Studies show a link between habitually high salt intake and higher blood pressure. But research indicates that limiting salt intake may reduce blood pressure–and reliance on antihypertensive medications. In the Trial of Nonpharmacologic Interventions in the Elderly, 975 men and women ages 60 to 80 with moderately high blood pressure controlled by medication were assigned to reduced sodium intake, weight loss, both, or usual care. After three months, most of the study participants could be taken off medication. Those who reduced their sodium intake were 31 percent less likely to have a subsequent relapse and require medication again.

The AHA recommends that you limit your sodium intake to 2,400 milligrams daily. That's less than a teaspoon of salt.

✔ *Monitor your alcohol intake.* Research indicates that alcohol raises blood pressure. One study, conducted by researchers at the University of California at San Diego, found that as few as two drinks a day produced a modest but consistent increase in both systolic and diastolic blood pressure. Men ages 35 and older who drank that amount were nearly twice as likely to have high blood pressure as men who didn't drink.

✔ *Reduce your caffeine intake.* Research on the relationship between caffeine and blood pressure is mixed: Some studies indicate that caffeine raises blood pressure; others do not. It is known, however, that an unaccustomed dose of caffeine can temporarily raise blood pressure.

✔ *Get enough calcium, magnesium, and potassium.* People with high blood pressure generally eat less calcium than people with normal blood pressure, and in one study, people with normal blood pressure who added 1,000 milligrams of calcium to their daily diets saw their diastolic blood pressure drop. Studies also show that getting enough magnesium, either through supplementation or diet, can help keep blood pressure low and that diets high in potassium help reduce high blood pressure–particularly high blood pressure connected to sodium intake. Foods rich in magnesium include whole grains, nuts, avocados, beans, and dark green leafy vegetables. Foods rich in calcium and potassium are listed on pages 50 and 51.

✔ *Follow the* **DASH** *diet.* The Dietary Approaches to Stop Hypertension Study (DASH), sponsored by the National Heart, Lung, and Blood Institute, tested the effects of three diets–a "typical American" control diet, a diet rich in fruits and vegetables, and a low-saturated-fat diet rich in fruits, vegetables, and low-fat dairy products (the DASH diet)–on people with high blood pressure. After eight weeks, all the people on the DASH diet experienced a drop in blood pressure. The DASH diet lowered average systolic blood pressure by 11.4 mm Hg and average diastolic blood pressure by 5.5 mm Hg–a reduction comparable to that achieved with antihypertensive drug therapy.

THE DASH DIET

The DASH diet is similar to the Dietary Guidelines for Americans, but it incorporates low-fat or nonfat dairy products and includes higher minimum servings of fruits and vegetables. Low in cholesterol, high in fiber, potassium, calcium, and magnesium, and moderately high in protein, the diet is a good guide to lowering your blood pressure and reducing your risk of hypertension, along with heart disease and stroke.

If you typically eat 2,000 calories per day, your diet should include these elements.

- Seven to eight servings of grains and grain products per day
- Four to five servings of vegetables per day
- Four to five servings of fruits per day
- Two to three servings of low-fat or nonfat dairy foods per day
- Two or fewer servings of meats, poultry, and fish per day
- Four to five servings of nuts, seeds, and legumes per week
- Limited servings of fats and sweets

Limit consumption of red meat.

If you're planning to throw some burgers on the grill or celebrate a special occasion in a fancy restaurant with a prime rib dinner, first consider your health. Red meat has been linked to cancer.

Although meats are good sources of protein and minerals such as iron and zinc, consumption of red meat has been linked to several cancers, notably those of the colon and prostate.

Researchers at Harvard Medical School and Brigham and Women's Hospital who studied 88,751 women found that those who ate beef, pork, or lamb as a main dish daily were two and one-half times more likely to develop colon cancer than those who ate red meat only once a month. And numerous studies indicate a relationship between prostate cancer and consumption of either fat or high-fat food, especially red meat, according to a review of epidemiologic studies reported in *Cancer Causes and Control*.

How red meat may promote cancer is still unknown. For prostate cancer, animal fat may be the major culprit. But even lean red meat appears to increase the risk of colon cancer. The cancer-causing effect of red meat could also be a result of carcinogens created when meat is cooked, points out Walter Willett, chair of the nutrition department at the Harvard School of Public Health. Cooked meats have been found to contain compounds, including a class of heterocyclic amines, that are carcinogenic in animals. These compounds are produced during high-temperature cooking such as broiling or frying, according to a study reported in *Environmental Health Perspectives*.

If you eat red meat, restrict it to less than 3 ounces a day (the size of a deck of cards), says an international group of experts, who also recommends only occasional consumption of cured, smoked meats and meat or fish grilled or broiled over direct flame.

 ## Include enough fiber in your diet.

Dietary fiber is primarily material from plant cell walls that your body cannot digest. Insoluble fiber (roughage) found in grains and vegetables does not dissolve in water. Soluble fiber, such as that found in oat bran, dissolves to form a gummy texture. Both provide important health benefits.

Reduced mortality from heart disease. Finnish researchers reported in the journal *Circulation* that men who ate the equivalent of three slices of rye bread—a good source of insoluble fiber—daily for six years cut their risk of dying from heart disease by 17 percent.

Lowered cholesterol. Soluble fiber binds with acids that are made from cholesterol in your liver, and then helps eliminate the acids. The liver responds by pulling more cholesterol from the blood, thereby lowering blood cholesterol levels.

Controlled diabetes. Harvard epidemiologists found that women who often ate low-fiber carbohydrates such as potatoes and refined flours during a six-year study were more than twice as likely to develop type 2 diabetes as were those who ate high-fiber cereals and brown rice.

Reduced risk of colorectal cancer. Insoluble fiber speeds digested food through the intestines, perhaps reducing the time the colon is in contact with carcinogens formed during digestion. It also forms a bulkier stool, which may dilute any cancerous substances. Further, a high-fiber diet tends to be low in fat, generally regarded to be another protector against cancer.

Lowered blood pressure. A high-fiber diet has been associated with lower blood pressure in some studies.

If you eat a typical American diet—about 10 to 15 grams a day—you probably need to double or triple the amount of fiber you consume. There's no RDA for fiber, but many experts recommend 20 to 35 grams a day.

Here are ways to add fiber to your diet.

✔ *Eat a variety of foods.* To get both soluble and insoluble fiber, add fruits, vegetables, cereals, and beans to your diet. Your best bets for insoluble fiber are whole wheat products, bran, and vegetables such as cauliflower, green beans, and potatoes. For soluble fiber, try dried beans and peas, oats, apples, oranges, and carrots.

✔ **Go whole grain.** When flour is milled, the outer layer of the grain (bran) and the inner section (germ) are removed. Unfortunately, this also removes fiber and nutrients.

✔ **Choose oatmeal.** Oats contain soluble fiber, which may help lower cholesterol levels and the risk of heart disease when they're included in a diet that is also low in saturated fat and cholesterol. In fact, the Food and Drug Administration has given certain oatmeal and oat bran manufacturers the green light to boast about the potential heart-healthy benefits of oats on their product labels. But you need about 1½ cups of cooked oatmeal daily to get the amount of soluble fiber necessary to lower your cholesterol. If you don't want to eat that much, add oats to pancakes, muffins, meatloaf, and breads.

 ## Avoid unhealthy food choices when eating out.

Americans are eating out more, and many of the places we rush to—such as McDonald's, where 7 percent of Americans eat on any given day, according to the *New York Times*—are not known for providing healthy foods. Considering the quantity of fat in fast foods such as hamburgers and fries, it's not surprising that research has found that regular fast food eaters are obese. A study published in the *American Journal of Public Health* connected obesity in women with a combination of frequent consumption of fast foods and television watching. Even a meal at more leisurely paced Chinese or Italian restaurants can provide unnecessary fat and calories. So choose carefully when you place your order.

✔ **Choose sandwiches wisely.** A McDonald's Big Mac has 530 calories and 28 grams of fat. A Burger King Whopper weighs in at 870 calories and 56 grams of fat. But a regular burger with a single patty has about 275 calories and 12 grams of fat. Likewise, while a fried chicken sandwich at Burger King tops out at 700 calories and 43 grams of fat, a grilled chicken breast sandwich typically has about 310 calories and 9 grams of fat.

✔ **Avoid supersize servings.** A typical restaurant meal averages 1,000 calories, according to the *Nutrition Action Healthletter.* And it can be double that amount when you add an appetizer or dessert.

✔ *Don't feel you have to finish everything on your plate.* Take some home for your next day's lunch or split an order with a friend.

✔ *Watch out for sauces and dressings.* Cream sauces, cheese sauces, mayonnaise, and salad dressings can seriously hike the fat content of accompanying foods. Ask for them on the side and use them in moderation.

Vitamins and Minerals

 Keep your eye on antioxidants.

You are probably familiar with antioxidants—molecules that neutralize dangerous free radicals. These highly unbalanced scavengers, which steal electrons from other molecules, promote oxidative chain reactions that are thought to damage the body's cells and lead to diseases such as cancer, heart disease, and arthritis, as well as damage the eyes and lungs. Antioxidants, including nutrients such as vitamin C, vitamin E, beta carotene, and selenium, neutralize free radicals and stop oxidative chain reactions, limiting cellular damage.

Evidence that these nutrients work to prevent or reduce the risk of disease is accumulating. More than 100 dietary studies have found that people who eat large amounts of fruits and vegetables with beneficial antioxidants have a reduced risk of cancer and heart disease. Antioxidant nutrients may also be an important key to longevity. An Italian study, published in the *Journal of the American Geriatric Society,* found that centenarians ate more vegetables and showed less oxidative stress—lower levels of fatty acids and glucose in their blood and lower levels of free radical activity—than younger study participants. Another study, by researchers at the National Institute on Aging, found that older people who took vitamin C and vitamin E supplements were 42 percent less likely to die of any cause during the three-year study period than were those who used neither supplement.

But the final word isn't in about antioxidants. Some studies have indicated that antioxidant supplements can actually have a negative effect on the body. The National Cancer Institute halted a major study ahead of schedule because study participants taking beta carotene supplements—almost all of whom were heavy smokers—were showing a higher risk of lung cancer and heart disease than those who weren't taking the supplements. And studies designed to isolate the effects of individual nutrients—often in supplement form—have not always echoed the findings of studies of foods.

It is possible that a combination of nutrients, or even other components in fruits and vegetables, are responsible for their beneficial effects. Flavonoids—phytochemical compounds that are found in tea, vegetables, fruits, and red wine—also have antioxidant properties. The exact role of these phytochemicals in promoting health is not yet known. Here are some of the diseases antioxidants may fight.

Atherosclerosis. In some studies, people with the highest intake of antioxidant vitamins have had fewer fatty deposits in their arteries.

Heart disease. Heart disease risk is lower in people who eat a lot of fruits and vegetables.

Stroke. Flavonoids and antioxidants may reduce the risk of stroke.

Cancer. Studies indicate that a diet containing five or more servings a day of fruits and vegetables cuts the risk of some cancers nearly in half.

Diabetes. Antioxidants may help reduce the risk of complications from diabetes, including kidney failure and death, according to research presented at the Experimental Biology '98 meeting.

Chronic obstructive pulmonary disease (COPD). Antioxidants may protect against COPD. In one study, the difference in lung function between study participants who consumed the most vitamin C, vitamin E, selenium, and beta carotene and those who consumed lower amounts was comparable to the difference between nonsmokers and pack-a-day smokers.

 Eat foods rich in beta carotene.

A high intake of beta carotene (which your body converts to vitamin A) is associated with a reduced risk of cancer. And foods—not supplements—are key. Beta-carotene-rich fruits and vegetables offer protection against cancer. Taken in supplement form, however, beta carotene may increase cancer risk–at least in some people.

In a review of 156 studies of fruit and vegetable intake and cancer risk, Gladys Block, Ph.D., professor of public health at the University of California at Berkeley, found that 128 studies support the protective effect of beta carotene-rich foods. But in one often-cited study, Finnish male smokers who took supplements containing 30 milligrams of beta carotene daily had a higher incidence of lung cancer than smokers who did not take the supplement.

A high dietary intake of beta carotene has also been linked to a reduced risk of heart disease. Two large Harvard University studies found that women with the highest intake of beta carotene were 22 percent less likely to develop heart disease than those with the lowest intake, and men with the highest beta carotene intake were 25 percent less likely to suffer heart attack, stroke, and other cardiovascular problems. However, studies have found that beta carotene supplements offer little or no reduction in cardiovascular disease risk.

Other possible health benefits from beta carotene include protecting the lungs against the damage caused by smoking and a reduced risk of rheumatoid arthritis.

Carrots, sweet potatoes, cantaloupes, leafy greens, squash, and apricots are good sources of beta carotene.

 Get enough vitamin C.

Like beta carotene, a high consumption of vitamin C is linked to a reduced risk of cancer. In an analysis of 90 studies that examined the effects of vitamin C on cancer, the University of California's Block found that high vitamin C intake correlated with lower cancer risk in three-quarters of the studies. Vitamin C's cancer-protective effects are attributed in part to its antioxidant status and in part to its role in maintaining and improving the functioning of the immune system.

Increased intake of vitamin C during infections and chronic illnesses may help speed recovery. Vitamin C may even protect the heart. The vitamin helps maintain the integrity of blood vessels and plays a role in metabolizing cholesterol. People with low vitamin C intake are often found to have high total cholesterol levels, and several studies have found that vitamin C lowers levels of dangerous LDL cholesterol and raises levels of beneficial HDL cholesterol. People with a low vitamin C intake or low levels of vitamin C in their blood also appear to be at increased risk of having high blood pressure. Finally, several recent studies indicate that vitamin C may help dilate blood vessels and help prevent blood from clotting, which can reduce the risk of heart attack and stroke.

Vitamin C can be found in citrus fruits, as well as strawberries, kiwifruits, cantaloupes, red and green bell peppers, broccoli, brussels sprouts, cabbages, peas, potatoes, asparagus, and dark green leafy vegetables.

How much vitamin C is enough? The RDA is 60 milligrams for men and women, and 100 milligrams for smokers, but many experts suggest a higher intake. Researchers at the National Institutes of Health, for instance, suggest that the RDA should be raised to 200 milligrams.

 Take vitamin E to prevent diseases.

Of all the antioxidants, vitamin E is the star. It holds the most promise for reducing the risk of heart disease, appears to boost the functioning of the immune system, and may reduce the risk of diabetic complications and some cancers and slow the progression of Alzheimer's disease.

So far, research indicates the following benefits from vitamin E.

Heart protection. Studies indicate that vitamin E protects LDL cholesterol from being oxidized, an early step in the development of atherosclerosis, and a growing number of studies indicate that vitamin E may reduce the severity or slow the progression of existing atherosclerosis. Vitamin E also decreases platelets' tendency to stick together and stick to other substances, thus reducing the risk of blood clots. Consequently, it may reduce the risk of heart disease, heart attack, and stroke.

Improved immune response. Vitamin E is essential for the normal functioning of the immune system and may even improve immune response. In studies of older individuals, the vitamin enhanced the function of beneficial T cells and increased the production of antibodies to various diseases.

Reduced diabetic complications. Studies have shown that blood glucose, insulin, and triglyceride levels fall in people with diabetes who take vitamin E supplements. Vitamin E also may protect the retina–the nerve layer at the back of the eye that senses light and helps send images to the brain–from damage.

Protection against some cancers, including those of the breast, colon, and prostate. In addition, several test-tube studies have found that vitamin E may help stop the proliferation of cancer cells and increase the effectiveness of cancer drugs. But there is also some evidence that vitamin E may encourage the spread of cancer in some people.

Delayed progression of Alzheimer's disease. In one study, Alzheimer's patients who took vitamin E experienced a delayed onset of the four important milestones of Alzheimer's disease progression. And in two studies of people with mild dementia, two common dietary supplements, vitamin E and ginkgo, delayed the progression of the disease in more than half of the study participants.

Vitamin E is found in oils, including soybean, cottonseed, peanut, corn, hazelnut, and sunflower, as well as in wheat germ, whole grain cereals, eggs, nuts, and fortified cereals.

The current RDA is 15 International Units (I.U.) for men and 12 I.U. for women, but most of the health benefits seen in studies have come from doses of 100 to 400 I.U. daily. If you have high blood pressure or are taking any blood-thinning medications such as warfarin (Coumadin), check with your physician before taking vitamin E supplements. Vitamin E may raise your risk of stroke if you have hypertension and may interfere with blood-thinning medications.

 Select selenium to reduce cancer risk.

Selenium is the latest antioxidant to make the headlines. In study reported in the *Journal of the American Medical Association* in 1996, people who took selenium supplements were 63 percent less likely to develop prostate cancer, 58 percent less likely to develop colorectal cancer, and 46 percent less likely to develop lung cancer than participants who took a placebo. This reinforces the findings of geographical studies, which have found that cancer rates are 10 percent higher in areas with selenium-poor soil (such as the Northwestern and Southeastern United States) than in areas with selenium-rich soil (such as the Midwestern United States).

Selenium is found in seafood, red meats such as liver and kidney, grains, eggs, chicken, garlic, and vegetables grown in selenium-rich soil. The RDA is 70 micrograms for men and 44 micrograms for women.

 ## Bone up on vitamin D.

More common than experts once believed, vitamin D deficiency has been dubbed a "silent epidemic." Between 30 and 40 percent of patients who are admitted to hospitals with hip fractures are deficient in vitamin D, according to a recent study published in the *Journal of the American Medical Association*. What do hip fractures have to do with longevity? Within three months of a hip fracture, between 10 and 20 percent of patients die as a result of complications. Another 20 percent die within the first year.

Vitamin D helps bone absorb calcium and phosphorus. The body makes the vitamin naturally when exposed to sunlight. As you get older, however, your capacity to make adequate amounts of the vitamin decreases. Try to get at least 15 minutes of sunlight daily—without sunblock—experts recommend.

For those who don't get a lot of sunlight, especially during winter months, milk and breakfast cereals are fortified with the vitamin. In northern winters (latitudes above Denver and Philadelphia), supplementation is recommended.

Vitamin D supplements must be taken carefully, however. Since the body stores vitamin D, excess vitamin D from supplements may lead to confusion, kidney stones, weak bones and muscles, and excessive bleeding. So stick to the recommendations. The National Academy of Sciences, which sets the RDAs and the new Dietary Reference

Intakes, has established an Adequate Intake of vitamin D at 200 I.U. per day for those under age 50; 400 I.U. for people ages 51 to 70; and 600 I.U. for those over age 70. To find out if you are deficient, especially if you are over age 50, have a blood test done in midwinter (in areas with less winter sun exposure).

 ## Get enough B vitamins to reduce heart disease risk.

The B vitamins work to help your body's cells produce energy. Increasing your intake of several of them—notably folic acid (a form of the B vitamin folate), vitamin B_6, and vitamin B_{12}—may reduce your risk of dying of heart disease.

In a study of more than 80,000 nurses, researchers found that those who had consumed at least 400 micrograms of folic acid daily had the lowest risk of dying from heart disease. The same study showed that those who consumed more than 3 milligrams of vitamin B_6 daily from supplements or food had the lowest rates of heart disease.

The heart-healthy benefits of folic acid and vitamin B_6 appear to come from their ability to lower blood levels of homocysteine, an amino acid that is found in higher levels in people with heart disease.

Since January 1998, the Food and Drug Administration has required enriched grains to be fortified with folic acid. Breakfast cereals, for example, now contain 25 percent of the RDA. Other good sources are spinach and navy beans. The RDA of folic acid is 400 micrograms for men and women and 600 micrograms for pregnant women.

Vitamin B_6 is also found in fortified cereals, as well as in meat, fish, poultry, potatoes and other starchy vegetables, and noncitrus fruits. The RDA is 1.3 milligrams for women and men ages 19 to 50; for women and men ages 51 and older, the RDAs are 1.5 milligrams and 1.7 milligrams, respectively.

Another important B vitamin is vitamin B_{12}, a vitamin whose levels begin declining as you age. Vitamin B_{12} is important in making blood cells and may also help lower blood levels of homocysteine. Breakfast cereals are fortified with the vitamin, which is also present in salmon, lean beef, yogurt, and shrimp. The RDA is 2.4 micrograms.

Mine your diet for necessary minerals.

Several other minerals besides selenium can help keep you healthy.

Potassium. An analysis of 33 studies reported in the *Journal of the American Medical Association* found that low potassium intake may lead to high blood pressure. Of the more than 2,500 patients in the studies, those who consumed an average of 2,340 milligrams of potassium a day experienced an average decrease in systolic blood pressure of 3.11 mm Hg and an average decrease in diastolic blood pressure of almost 2 mm Hg. Other studies have shown that eating a single extra serving of a food rich in potassium every day may cut the risk of fatal stroke by between 25 and 40 percent.

There is no RDA for potassium, but the American Dietetic Association reports that some experts recommend 3,500 milligrams daily to reduce blood pressure. (People with kidney failure or on medications that interfere with potassium excretion should not increase potassium to control hypertension because too much potassium in the body can be toxic.) Potassium is found in fruits and vegetables and their juices. Good sources include bananas, prunes, raisins, avocados, potatoes, and beet greens.

Calcium. Most Americans consume less than the recommended amount of calcium, which is important to maintain bone strength, especially in postmenopausal women. Recent studies have also shown that calcium may reduce colon cancer risk, and the calcium consumed in food has been found to reduce formation of kidney stones.

Be sure you know when and how best to take the mineral. Your body's calcium absorption is affected by other nutrients. If you don't get enough vitamin D, for example, your body may not absorb and use calcium correctly. A diet high in sodium and animal protein also decreases calcium absorption, while intake of antacids (except calcium carbonate tablets) increases loss of the mineral through urination. On the other hand, if you consume calcium with iron, your iron absorption can be decreased by as much as 50 percent. If you take a calcium supplement, take it between meals to avoid such interactions.

Good food sources of calcium include calcium-fortified orange juice, low-fat dairy products, dark green vegetables, canned fish, legumes, and nuts. The National Academy of Sciences has established an Adequate Intake of 1,000 milligrams per day for adults up to age 50 and 1,200 milligrams per day for those ages 51 and older. The National Institutes of Health recommends a daily intake of 1,200 milligrams for adults and 1,500 milligrams for postmenopausal women.

Iron. Adolescents and premenopausal women may have iron deficiencies, but the rest of the population may be getting too much iron, according to the U.S. Department of Agriculture. This high-iron diet can have negative health effects. True, younger women lose iron through menstruation, but men under age 50 are five times more likely than women to show symptoms of hemochromatosis, a deadly genetic disease that causes the body to store too much iron. The disease affects 1.5 million Americans and can lead to diabetes and heart and liver damage. The latest findings point to iron as a possible contributor to increased risk of heart disease.

The RDA of iron is 10 milligrams for men and for women over age 50 and 15 milligrams for women ages 11 to 50. Iron can be found in meat, fish, eggs, and whole grains.

 Choose vitamin and mineral supplements wisely.

Supplements are not substitutes for a balanced diet. They don't provide important disease-fighting phytochemicals (plant-based substances) found only in fruits and vegetables. In general, the American diet is varied and inexpensive enough to provide all the nutrients you need to live a long life. But you may need to take supplements of nutrients such as vitamin E to achieve the additional health benefits seen in studies. If you do decide to supplement your vitamin and mineral intake, keep in mind these suggestions from the American Dietetic Association.

✔ **Go generic.** Generic products may not be packaged as prettily, but they pack the same nutritional punch as heavily advertised name brands.

✔ **Don't fear synthetics.** A man-made vitamin or mineral is generally as effective and safe as a "natural" formulation and usually a lot cheaper. The natural supplements, extracted from plants, are usually called phytonutrients. There is little evidence that these plant-derived supplements are better, however. Thousands of plants can be used, and no one knows what the best ones are for individual vitamins.

✔ *Check the expiration date.*

✔ *Ignore extras.* Extra ingredients such as choline, herbs, or amino acids add cost, but no nutritional value.

Hormones and Nutritional Supplements

 Know the role of hormone replacements.

Although the search for the mythical fountain of youth ended centuries ago, the search for a magic potion to counteract the aging process and extend life continues today. Hormone supplements ranging from estrogen and testosterone to DHEA and melatonin are among the latest of these magic potions. Contrary to popular claims, though, none of these hormones has been shown to prevent or reverse aging, according to the National Institute on Aging (NIA).

Although some hormones, such as estrogen and testosterone, do have proven health benefits and research may ultimately reveal important health benefits from others, the NIA urges consumers to use caution in taking hormone supplements to combat aging. Hormone supplements are powerful chemicals that enter the bloodstream and travel throughout the body. Tiny amounts may have far-reaching effects, and unsupervised use of any hormone supplement, in any amount, can lead to health problems. Three of the "antiaging hormones"–estrogen, testosterone, and human growth hormone– are available only by prescription, but DHEA and melatonin are available over the counter and are unregulated by the Food and Drug Administration.

Here are some of the hormones being sold to combat aging and what they can and cannot do.

Estrogen. This female hormone is widely prescribed to postmenopausal women to relieve menopausal symptoms such as hot flashes and vaginal dryness and to counteract conditions such as heart disease and osteoporosis that are related to the decline in estrogen.

Estrogen helps bones absorb calcium and helps retard bone-thinning during postmenopausal years. It also reduces blood levels of harmful LDL cholesterol and increases levels of beneficial HDL cholesterol, offering protection from atherosclerosis and heart disease. In addition, studies indicate that estrogen may help reduce the risk of Alzheimer's disease, diabetes, and colorectal cancer. But it is known to increase the risk of endometrial cancer if not given in conjunction with the hormone progesterone. Some studies indicate that it may also increase the risk of breast cancer.

Testosterone. This male hormone, which is normally prescribed to men with testosterone deficiency, is used to treat reduced libido in postmenopausal women and has recently been touted as an anti-aging supplement for men. Although research indicates that testosterone supplementation may help improve bone mass, muscle mass, and strength in older men and could have positive effects on mood, cognition, and sexual function in some men, a report in the *Journal of Andrology* concludes that questions remain about the magnitude and longevity of the beneficial effects, whether only certain subgroups of men would benefit from therapy, and the long-term effects, particularly as they relate to heart disease and prostate cancer.

DHEA. Dehydroepiandrosterone, or DHEA, is a "mother" hormone, which means that the body uses it to make testosterone and estrogen. Because levels of DHEA fall steadily with age, some researchers have theorized that keeping DHEA levels at their youthful high could stave off heart disease, cancer, diabetes, impotence, memory loss, and a host of other ailments associated with aging. Some animal studies support this theory, but there is very little solid research in humans. Studies of old mice indicate that DHEA may boost immune function, prevent some types of cancer, and delay osteoporosis, and a study using rabbits indicates that DHEA might counter atherosclerosis. One small study in humans showed increased feelings of well-being in older people who took DHEA, but no large, long-term studies have been completed. Even though small doses appear to have no adverse effects, DHEA may affect the body in some of the same ways as testosterone and estrogen. DHEA has been known to cause irreversible masculinization—body hair, deepening voice—and premature menopause in women, and some experts believe it could increase the risk of prostate cancer in men.

Human growth hormone. This naturally occurring hormone, which like DHEA and other hormones declines as we age, was recently approved as a treatment for short children with a growth hormone deficiency. It has been prescribed by some "antiaging" clinics to retard aging, but little is known about its use or safety in adults or people without deficiencies.

Melatonin. More than 20 million Americans take melatonin to fight insomnia, prevent jet lag, battle cancer, rejuvenate the sex life, and slow aging. But little solid evidence backs up these claims. This hormone, released into the bloodstream by the pineal gland between dusk and 2 A.M. and 4 A.M., may play a role in many body processes. According to the *Mayo Clinic Health Letter,* the blood vessels, ovaries, gastrointestinal system, and brain all have cells that are specially equipped to use melatonin. But to date, most is known about its role in initiating the changes in your body that make you feel ready for sleep.

 Educate yourself about herbs, amino acids, and other supplements.

Hormones are not the only "antiaging" supplements on the market. A number of herbal remedies, amino acids, and other supplements are also being touted as life extenders. These include the herbs ginkgo biloba, ginseng, and St. John's wort, the amino acids glutathione and L-phenylalanine, and antioxidants such as pycnogenol, superoxide dismutase (SOD), and coenzyme Q_{10}.

There is no question that herbs have a variety of therapeutic actions in the body: Many modern medicines are based on herbal remedies. Amino acids, the building blocks of proteins, also have specific bodily functions. Further, research supports the theory that oxidative damage contributes to aging, and antioxidants may help counter heart disease, some cancers, cataracts, and other problems of aging. But caution is warranted in relying on these substances to turn back the clock. Although these substances are available over the counter, they do have action in the body, and taking them in excess or taking them in combination with other supplements or medications may prove dangerous. Therefore, you should check with your doctor before trying any of these supplements.

Antiaging Supplements

SUPPLEMENT	USE	CAUTIONS
Herbs		
Echinacea	Boosts immune function; has anti-inflammatory and antiviral properties	Do not use if you are allergic to plants in the sunflower family.
Ginkgo biloba	Improves brain function; improves circulation; useful for depression and memory loss	Do not use if you have a bleeding disorder or are pregnant or nursing.
Ginseng	Boosts immune function; increases circulation; increases energy	Do not use if you have low blood sugar, hypertension, or heart disorders.
St. John's wort	May boost immunity against infection; useful for depression	Be aware that it may cause heightened sensitivity to sun.
Amino Acids		
Glutathione	Improves mental function; improves mood; has antioxidant properties	
L-Phenylalanine	Promotes alertness	Do not use if you are pregnant or nursing, suffer from panic attacks, or have diabetes or hypertension.
Antioxidants		
Coenzyme Q_{10}	Improves circulation; protects the heart	
Pycnogenol	Has potent antioxidant properties	
Superoxide dismutase (SOD)	Neutralizes the free radical superoxide; reduces cellular destruction	Be aware that supplements have no effect on the body; they are broken up during digestion.

3 ■ Injury Prevention

There are approximately 92,000 accidental deaths in the United States each year, making accidents the fifth leading cause of death. Of all accidents, motor vehicle crashes are the leading cause of unintentional injury and death. In 1997, 42,065 people lost their lives, according to the National Highway Traffic Safety Administration. For about 24,000 Americans a year, the home environment is as dangerous as the highway. Unsafe stairways or bathrooms, fires that race through the house, and even carbon monoxide leaks are responsible for many deadly accidents in the home.

Other household dangers also lurk, including the food we eat and the water we drink. The Environmental Protection Agency reported several years ago that the drinking water in 819 cities—supplying water to more than 30 million Americans—had excess levels of lead. But the environment outside the home isn't necessarily safer. In 1997, 100 people were felled by lightning strikes, and 900 people lost their lives in bicycle accidents.

In many cases, fatal accidents can be avoided with a little extra effort or foresight. Accident prevention can make a major difference in your life span. According to the National Center for Health Statistics, if all the people who were killed in accidents had somehow been able to avoid the situation that caused the fatality, they would have added an estimated 23 to 38 years to their lives.

Home Safety

 Don't fall for it.

Falls are the second leading cause of preventable accidental death in the United States. And the older you get, the more likely a fall will be fatal. Roughly 5,000 people over age 75 die every year as a result of falls, mostly in their homes. When older people fall, they are more likely to sustain the kind of injury—such as a broken hip—that can lead to a major health problem. In fact, for those Americans who have the brittle bone disease osteoporosis, complications from fractures lead to approximately 40,000 deaths annually. Here are some suggestions to reduce your chances of taking that first fatal misstep.

✔ *Make sure hallways and stairs are well lit.*

✔ *Keep night-lights burning in hallways and bathrooms.*

✔ *Make sure stairway railings and the steps themselves are secure.*

✔ *Keep stairs and walkways clear.*

✔ *Use contrasting colors or plant arrangements to draw attention to short flights of stairs.*

✔ *Don't run electrical cords through traffic areas.*

✔ *Secure area or throw rugs to the floor with double-sided adhesive tape.* Replace worn runners on stairs and use only bath mats with nonslip bottoms.

✔ *Put nonslip appliqués in your bathtub.* And install a grab bar in the bathtub or shower.

✔ *When purchasing new carpet, choose a shorter pile such as Berber.* You're less likely to catch a heel in the fibers of shorter piles.

 Take precautions to avoid fires.

Every year, fires in the home kill about 4,000 Americans. Most people don't die of burns, but of the smoke and toxic gases they inhale when a fire consumes everything in its path. You can protect yourself and your family from fires, however, if you take these precautions.

✔ **Install smoke detectors.** Most home fires happen between 10 P.M. and 6 A.M. while the family is asleep. That's why smoke detectors are so important. Install them on every level of your house. If you have a smoker in the house, it may be advisable to install one in his or her bedroom. Careless smoking is the main cause of fire deaths in the home. Smoke detectors should be mounted on ceilings, four inches from a wall, or high on walls, four inches from the ceiling. The devices should be replaced every 10 years.

✔ **Make sure your smoke detectors work.** A third of all smoke alarms are useless because the batteries are dead. Check the batteries the first week of every month by depressing the test button. Replace the batteries as soon as they emit the "beeping" that shows they are running down–or at least once a year. You can also use lithium batteries that last for years or have the alarms permanently wired in.

✔ **Keep fire extinguishers handy.** Multipurpose Class ABC extinguishers are best for home use, the National Safety Council advises. Check gauges regularly and have extinguishers refilled when the indicators read "recharge."

✔ **Make a plan.** Develop a home evacuation plan and practice it with your family. Identify two exits and make sure everyone knows where they are.

Here are several helpful tips to reduce the likelihood of a fire in your home.

✔ **Don't use space heaters,** which, despite new safety measures, still may overheat.

✔ **Don't store propane gas tanks in garages.** Gas fumes may escape and be ignited when you flick the light switch. Store them outside, away from buildings but protected from the elements.

✔ **Don't run electrical cords under rugs,** where they may overheat. And replace all old or damaged electrical outlets with modern three-pronged ones that provide grounding, suggests the National Fire Protection Association.

Don't be shocked—protect yourself from electricity.

Ben Franklin got a bit of a jolt the day he flew a kite into the stormy Philadelphia sky. He lived to tell the tale, but others who have come into direct contact with electricity have not been so lucky. Hundreds of Americans die every year as a result of electrocutions in their own homes. Yet it's easy to protect yourself from electrical shock.

If your home is more than 10 years old, you may want to have an electrician install ground fault circuit interrupters (GFCIs). Building codes require them in new homes, but GFCIs didn't exist when many older homes were built. GFCIs monitor electricity flowing through your home's system. When an individual GFCI senses a disruption in the circuitry—including a disruption caused by electricity flowing through a human being—it automatically turns off the power. GFCIs should be installed wherever appliances come into contact with water, counsels the National Electrical Safety Foundation.

Here are more ways to make your home less shocking.

✔ *Replace appliance electrical cords that are darkened or frayed.*

✔ *Don't overload sockets or outlets with extension cords.*

✔ *Never use electrical appliances near bathtubs, sinks, and pools.*

✔ *Don't use electrical tools outside when there is early morning dew or if it is raining.* And make sure any extension cords you use outside are for outdoor use.

 ## Don't give carbon monoxide emissions permission.

Every year, about 100,000 people are poisoned by carbon monoxide (CO), and about 200 people die of carbon monoxide poisoning associated with home fuel-burning heating equipment, according to the Consumer Product Safety Commission. Yet almost all deaths from CO can be avoided.

Carbon monoxide is found whenever a fuel such as wood, charcoal, natural gas, gasoline, oil, or kerosene is burned without enough oxygen. When you breathe in the gas, the carbon monoxide accumulates and binds to your red blood cells, crowding out oxygen. Initial symptoms may be weakness, confusion, and dizziness.

Here's what experts say will lower your risk of being poisoned by carbon monoxide.

✔ *Install a carbon monoxide detector outside your bedroom area.* Similar to smoke detectors, carbon monoxide detectors beep when they detect a leak. Make sure the detector is Underwriters Laboratory rated. If you hear the detector beep, leave the area and seek medical attention immediately. Tell the health care provider you may have been exposed to carbon monoxide.

✔ *Have your fuel-burning appliances checked for leaks.* Streaks of carbon or soot around appliances or stains on flue pipes may indicate a problem. And never bring a charcoal grill indoors, even into the garage, after you've recently used it. Although the fire may appear to be out, coals can still emit dangerous carbon monoxide that builds up in the confined area.

✔ *Don't let a car idle with the garage doors shut.* Always drive into the garage front first to allow the gas to dissipate through the garage door opening.

✔ *During winter, watch for CO accumulations inside the car.* If you get stuck in a snowdrift and need to run the engine to keep warm while awaiting help, lower the windows a little. The fresh air will keep you alert—and alive. And keep the area around the exhaust pipe clear.

✔ *In summer, make sure you have carbon monoxide detectors on your boat.* Recreational boaters may be at risk for accidental carbon monoxide poisoning even if their boats are working perfectly, according to a study reported in the *Journal of the American Medical Association.* Exhaust from the engine is the most common culprit, but exhaust from water heaters, space heaters, and generators also contributes.

✔ *When using gasoline-powered tools in buildings or semi-enclosed spaces, make sure the area is well ventilated.* About 10 percent of all carbon monoxide poisoning is believed to result from using these tools in enclosed spaces. Use the "buddy" system when working with a potential CO generator; each person should be on guard against the initial symptoms, which include disorientation and loss of consciousness.

Reduce your risk of radon exposure.

Every year, lung cancer kills as many as 14,000 Americans who neither smoke nor are regularly exposed to secondhand smoke. According to the Surgeon General, radon is the leading cause of lung cancer among nonsmokers and the second leading cause of lung cancer among smokers. In the United States, about one house in a thousand probably has unacceptably high radon levels–above 20 picocuries per liter of air, according to the Environmental Protection Agency (EPA). The good news is that these houses cluster in certain geographic areas, making it easier to detect radon.

Radon is a naturally occurring gas produced when radium and uranium decay in rocks and soil. Radon can flow from the earth through cracks in a foundation or walls, spaces around sump pumps and pipes, and through construction joints. As radon decays, it attaches to dust particles that can lodge in the lungs and eventually may cause cancer.

Here's how to find out if radon lurks in your basement and what to do if it does.

✔ *Contact your local health department.* Staff can tell you if radon is likely to be a problem in your area. Your local EPA office is also likely to be aware of the radon risk where you live. For a list of state radon agency phone numbers, check out the EPA Web site at www.epa.gov/radonpro/contacts.html.

✔ *Get an EPA-approved test kit.* Some health departments make these available for a reasonable fee. You can also find kits in hardware stores for $10 to $30. The test kit includes a charcoal canister that absorbs the gas and begins to register the level of radon within a few days. Keep in mind that levels vary, even from day to day. Radon is usually more concentrated in winter months when more of it gets trapped in a weather-sealed house. "Electret" and "alpha-track" detectors, which measure levels for up to three months, give you a better idea of whether you have a problem than do short-term testing canisters, which only measure radon for a few days.

✔ *If radon is found, consult an EPA-certified radon removal expert who can help you evaluate your home.* A professionally installed removal system costs from $800 to $1,500, depending on the your house. Things you can do yourself include installing window fans to vent the radon outside and tightly sealing all openings in the basement where the radon might be entering. If you or someone else in your family smokes, you should know that experts say the combination of radon and smoking is especially deadly.

 ## Don't breathe in secondhand smoke.

Nonsmokers who live with smokers have an increased risk of dying from the secondhand smoke. To ensure that both you and your smoking cohabitant live long and prosper, encourage and help him or her stop smoking. (See page 94.) If smoking cessation is not an option, try to limit your exposure to the smoke by asking the smoker to smoke only in certain rooms you don't enter or, better yet, outdoors.

Approximately one-fifth of the 177,000 lung cancers diagnosed each year are the result of breathing in environmental tobacco smoke for at least one accumulated hour weekly. Secondhand smoke accounts for 3,000 deaths a year, according to the Environmental Protection Agency.

In addition, secondhand smoke contributes to atherosclerosis, which increases the risk of heart attack and stroke. One study found that progression of atherosclerosis increased 20 percent more in those exposed to cigarette smoke than in those not exposed. This makes being exposed to secondhand smoke one-third as likely to speed up atherosclerosis as directly puffing on cigarettes.

Here's what other studies have found out about the risks of secondhand smoke.

■ Nonsmokers who live with heavy smokers have a higher risk of heart attack than those who live in a smoke-free environment, according to a study reported in the *Journal of the American College of Cardiology*. The risk is greater for men than women. Nonsmoking male members of smoking households saw their risk of heart attack increase 92 percent; nonsmoking female members of smoking households saw their risk increase 50 percent.

■ Both active and passive smoking cause stiffening of the aorta, the main artery that exits the heart to supply blood to the rest of the body. The stiffness forces the heart to work harder to pump blood.

■ Nonsmokers who spend as little as half an hour in a smoke-filled room suffer from a drop in their blood levels of healthy antioxidants such as vitamin C. The environmental smoke may also encourage low-density lipoprotein, the "bad" cholesterol, to be deposited in arteries.

Food Poisoning and Water Contamination

 Prepare food carefully to avoid dangerous pathogens.

Although the U.S. food supply is generally safe, food poisoning is on the rise, in part because of the growth of national distribution. National distribution makes it harder to track foods and stop sales when a problem occurs. When a nationally distributed brand of ice cream was contaminated by the *Salmonella enteritidis* bacterium, for example, it sickened about 250,000 people throughout the United States before the pattern in illnesses was noticed. *Escherichia coli* (*E. coli*) has shown up in apple juice and has also caused widespread outbreaks from undercooked hamburger meat. And *Salmonella* has been found in eggs nationwide and also in about 16 percent of the chicken sold in stores.

Whereas most reactions to *Salmonella* are essentially harmless gastrointestinal symptoms, *E. coli* infection can lead to sudden kidney failure, stroke, and brain damage, especially in the elderly.

In addition, new pathogens are cropping up in foods. Formerly uncommon, the *Campylobacter* bacterium now is thought to be the most likely source of foodborne bacterial infections in the United States–responsible for about 4 million cases each year. *Campylobacter* can cause a serious blood infection in people with diabetes or cancer and can lead to heart valve infection and meningitis. And uncooked seafood contaminated with *Salmonella*, *Campylobacter*, or viruses such as hepatitis A can be especially dangerous to those with liver, kidney, or gastrointestinal disease.

All told, about 4,500 people die every year of conditions caused by bad food. Fortunately, many cases of food poisoning can be avoided. About 85 percent of all outbreaks are a result of mishandling food—in food establishments or at home. The tips that follow will help you pay careful attention in preparing what you eat and making safe choices in restaurants.

✔ *Make sure that foods from animal sources (meats, dairy products, eggs) are pasteurized or properly cooked.* Make sure cooked meats are gray or brown—not pink inside—and juices run clear. To be extra safe, use a meat thermometer. Hamburger meat should be cooked to an internal temperature of 160°F to kill *E. coli* bacteria. Eggs should be cooked until the whites are set and the yolks begin to thicken.

✔ *Keep utensils (knives, cutting boards, bowls) you used to prepare foods from animal sources separate from other foods.* Wash the utensils thoroughly with soap and water after use. You can sanitize a cutting board with 2 teaspoons of liquid bleach mixed with 1 quart of water.

✔ *Keep foods from animal sources refrigerated.* Bacteria need time to grow into the vast numbers that can sicken people. They begin to grow to dangerous levels in food left unrefrigerated for one hour outdoors or two hours indoors. Eggs should always be refrigerated until just before you use them. If you need to let eggs approach room temperature when you are baking, take them out 20 minutes before mixing.

✔ *Don't prepare food if you are sick with symptoms that include vomiting or diarrhea.*

✔ *Wash your hands with soap and water both before and after preparing food.*

✔ *Wash the food thermometer with soap and hot water after you've used it on meat.*

✔ *Keep fresh shellfish (clams, oysters, crabs, lobsters) alive in the refrigerator until you cook them.* Discard any that are dead (the shells of dead clams and oysters will be open). Buy shellfish only from markets that use shellfish harvested from state-approved waters.

Up to 16 percent of chickens may be contaminated with *Salmonella enteritidis*. Most of the hens infected with the bacteria, which they pass into their eggs, are in the Northeast. But hens in other parts of the country also are showing the infection.

To avoid getting sick from poultry, heed the following advice.

✔ *Buy chicken that is well wrapped, with no leakage from the package.* Make sure it is cool to the touch.

✔ *Never thaw chicken on a countertop.* Thaw it in the refrigerator, instead, being careful to keep the blood from contaminating other refrigerated foods. This goes for the Thanksgiving turkey too. It will take about a day to thaw a 4-pound bird, so plan ahead.

✔ *Cook chicken thoroughly.* The inside meat temperature should be at least 180°F.

✔ *Never place cooked and raw chicken on the same preparation surface.*

✔ *Don't use eggs that have cracked or dirty shells.*

 Don't let eating out make you sick.

Protect yourself in a restaurant or at a celebration by following these suggestions.

✔ *When at informal functions such as church picnics and PTA dinners, avoid egg-based foods such as potato salad and coleslaw.* *Salmonella* bacteria begin to multiply dangerously after an hour. And you may not know how long ago the food was prepared or when it left the refrigerator.

✔ *Make sure meats and poultry are cooked thoroughly when you receive your food.* Send undercooked food back for more cooking.

✔ *Avoid restaurant dishes that use raw eggs such as hollandaise sauce or Caesar salad dressing.* Because restaurants prepare foods in large quantities, they often break as many as 500 eggs at a time to make a "pool" that is used throughout the day. This allows one infected egg to contaminate the entire batch.

Test your tap water.

No one knows exactly how many people get sick from drinking tap water that's been contaminated with bacteria, but experts agree the number is substantial. The U.S. drinking water supply is the safest in the world, but animal wastes, agricultural runoff, and industrial pollution can all add contaminants to your drinking water.

If you have municipal water, your local health department and water utility will let you know if there's a problem—if they know. But if you're one of the millions of Americans who get their water from private wells, you are responsible for making sure your water is safe. Private wells, especially those that are 50 feet deep or less, may be contaminated with *E. coli* bacteria, pesticides, and anemia-causing nitrates. Protect yourself by following these tips.

✔ *Have your water tested at least once a year for bacteria, radon, and inert chemicals such as arsenic* if your water comes from a well or other groundwater source.

✔ *Test your water for organic chemicals such as nitrates and benzenes* if you live in an industrialized area.

✔ *Test your water for lead contamination* if your home is 20 years or older. The pipes may be lead pipes or have lead in the solder used for joints.

For testing, call your local health department. Or call these mail-order companies for test kits: National Testing Laboratories, 800-458-333; or Suburban Water Testing Laboratories, 800-433-6595. You can also visit Suburban's Web site at www.h20test.com.

 ## Select the right water filtration system.

Selling bogus water-treatment devices to uneducated consumers is the newest scam of unscrupulous salespeople. To avoid being taken for a ride, choose a reputable dealer and a treatment system certified by the National Sanitation Foundation (NSF). NSF-certified devices list the pollutants they remove. Compare the treatment system list with your water test results before treatment to be sure that any filtration system you use eliminates the specific contaminants found in your water.

Most houseware departments sell specially designed water pitchers with activated carbon (charcoal) filters. Other versions attach to the kitchen faucet. Most activated carbon filters can remove bad tastes, odors, and organic compounds, including pesticides, chloroform, and solvents. However, they won't remove bacteria, nitrates, sodium, or fluoride, and most won't trap heavy metals such as lead. To get the lead out, you need a lead filter cartridge. If the system you've chosen claims to remove lead, look for the Underwriters Laboratories seal to back up the claim. And change the filters frequently. If you don't, they fill up with the very contaminants you are trying to avoid.

For more thorough filtering, a reverse osmosis filtering system eliminates almost all contaminants, including lead, arsenic, asbestos, parasite cysts, and nitrates from fertilizers. Found in home supply stores, these devices are installed under sinks or in nearby spaces and collect water in tanks for later use. They cost several hundred dollars, however, usually require professional installation, and require periodic replacements of the cartridges that collect the contaminants.

 Beware of the contents of bottled water.

Expensive bottled water isn't necessarily pure. The Food and Drug Administration has established standards for bottled water, but experts say that lack of enforcement means bottled waters have been shown to contain anything from pesticides to chemical solvents. In addition, three-quarters of the companies that bottle and sell water simply use local tap water. To protect yourself, find out what's really in the water you're buying.

Spring water. This is groundwater that comes to the surface. If the groundwater is contaminated by industrial and agricultural sources, the water may be full of potentially harmful pollutants such as bacteria or industrial chemicals. The plastic jugs that hold the water can also be a problem. Bacteria can cling to their sides, and sometimes chemical solvents from the plastics leach into the water. To find pure spring water, look for a local bottling company located in a nonindustrial area. Bottles should say "natural spring water." And ask the bottler if steps have been taken to prevent contamination from the plastic containers. The answer should tip you off to how well they are handling the problem.

Sparkling water (any carbonated water). This water often has added salt that can be harmful to people with diabetes and high blood pressure. Check the label before you buy.

Seltzer (filtered, carbonated tap water). Seltzer is a good choice for those avoiding salt, but it often has added sugar. Carefully read the ingredients listed on the bottle.

Travel Safety

 Buy a car that's "crashworthy."

A well-designed vehicle is one of the most important factors that can save your life in an accident. Crashworthiness means a strong driver/passenger compartment–called the safety cage–and front and rear ends that absorb crashes–the crush zone. The crush zone must be designed to keep damage away from the safety cage. The larger the crush zone, the more likely you are to survive an accident.

Here are points to consider when choosing a safe car.

Four door vs. two-door. Four-door vehicles are structurally stronger than two-door vehicles because they have heavy steel "B" pillars between the front and back doors.

Large vs. small. Size and weight matter. Small cars have three times the occupant death rate of bigger cars, mostly because larger cars have longer crush zones. In a head-on collision–the most common kind of any collision, according to the National Highway Traffic Safety Administration–the bigger vehicle will drive the smaller one backward, reducing some of its own crash force but adding to the smaller vehicle's deadly direction.

On the other hand, bigger vehicles exert more force on occupants when they are involved in a single-vehicle collision with an immobile object such as a stone wall.

Of course, you can't predict what kind of an accident you may encounter. But if you drive mostly on suburban or country roads and feel you are more likely to come bumper to tree than bumper to bumper, you may want to consider a smaller car.

Individual differences. Not all cars are made the same. Some have crush zones that are too stiff or short, and some vehicles' safety cages are inadequate to protect occupants. The Insurance Institute for Highway Safety evaluates cars for safety in a 40 mph front-end crash, including an overall rating on how well the vehicle protects people during a crash. According to the institute, the safest 1998 model midsize four-door cars—their "best picks"—are the Ford Taurus, Mercury Sable, Volkswagen Passat, Volvo 850/S70, and Toyota Camry; the safest 1998 model small car is the Volkswagen New Beetle. For a complete list of ratings, contact the institute at 1005 N. Glebe Rd., Suite 800, Arlington, VA 22201; 703-247-1500 or visit their Web site at www.highwaysafety.org.

 Learn the pros and cons of air bags.

Air bags are estimated to have saved more than 2,500 lives. But since 1990, they have also contributed to 113 deaths, the majority in people of smaller stature—namely, women and children—who are more likely to be injured by the bags' 200 mph impact. Safety experts have found that most deaths from air bags occurred when passengers were too close to the air bag when it inflated. That included reaching down to pick up a tissue off the floor or adjusting the radio just before a crash.

Now, the National Highway Traffic Safety Administration (NHTSA) has ruled that the devices, mandated in all 1998 and future models, can be turned off. You need to install a special switch to do so and to obtain permission from the NHTSA by demonstrating you have small stature or a medical condition such as osteoporosis that makes the bags dangerous. Before you decide to be without an air bag's proven safety, however, consider these points.

■ If you're petite, the best way to avoid an air bag-related fatality is to allow at least 10 inches between the air bag cover and your breastbone. You may need to slide the seat back to do this. You can also can recline your seat backward a notch or change the steering wheel position. If this makes it difficult to see the road, try sitting on a small pillow.

■ Cars built in 1998 and after have what automakers call "Generation II" air bags, which are slower-inflating air bags with speeds reduced by about 25 percent. And now, automakers have begun to put air bags in the dashboard–rather than the steering column–where they will be slowed down by hitting the windshield before they hit you.

You may also want to choose a new car with side air bags designed to protect the chest during a side-impact collision. Not surprisingly, cars with this option are among the priciest. If you can afford to spend as much as $30,000 for a car, however, the side air bags may be a worthwhile investment. Even some less expensive models have them, including the 1998 Chevrolet Prizm. In addition, Ford has said it will phase side air bags into all models by 2001, starting with the 1999 Mercury Cougar, the 1999 Ford Windstar minivan, and the 2000 Lincoln LS sedan.

Cars with side air bags available in 1998 and later models include Audi (except the A6 wagon and Cabrio); BMW (except some 3-series); Cadillac (except Catera and Eldorado); Chevrolet Venture and Prizm; Infiniti I30 and Q45; Jaguar XJ-8; Lexus ES/GS/LS; all Mercedes models; Nissan Maxima; Oldsmobile Silhouette minivans; Pontiac Trans Sport; Porsche Boxster; Toyota Avalon, Camry, and Corolla; Volkswagen Passat; and all Volvos, according to the Insurance Institute for Highway Safety.

 ## Use antilock brakes correctly.

Beginning in the early 1990s, automakers began to equip cars with a safety feature that avoids the problem of brakes that lock up in an emergency–the antilock braking system (ABS). But you may need to "brake" old habits to use ABS safely.

An antilock braking system pumps automatically to avoid dangerous brake lockup and to help you maintain control on slippery surfaces. The brakes pump up to speeds of 20 times per second. Unfortunately, antilock brakes haven't been proven to reduce crashes, says the NHTSA. In fact, cars with antilock brakes are *more* likely to be in crashes in which a car runs off the road and hits another object or rolls over. It's not known why this is the case, but automakers suspect drivers with antilock brakes may not know how to use them correctly.

If you have antilock brakes, your best bet is to read your owner's manual to find out the manufacturer's suggestions for use. Keep in mind that if you've been taught to pump the brakes on slippery roads to avoid skidding, you will now have to learn not to do that. ABS is activated by hard, continuous pressure. Hold your foot down until you feel the vibration that indicates the brakes are working.

You may want to go for some test runs in a deserted parking lot with puddles or light snow to get a feel for how they work.

 ## Stow objects safely to avoid killer cargo.

Inside a moving vehicle, loose personal items can become deadly projectiles. If you're like most people, you probably get in your car and plunk down your briefcase, handbag, or shopping bags on the seat next to you. If you've been shopping, a bag with silk lingerie shouldn't cause much of a problem. But if you just bought some tools or have a stuffed briefcase or laptop computer resting in the passenger seat, you can be at risk. When objects like these become airborne, they can injure or kill car occupants.

The solution is simple. Get in the habit of putting any heavy items, including your briefcase or computer, in the trunk. You can tuck your handbag under the seat, where it's less likely to become airborne.

 ## Restrain yourself in the car.

When an accident happens, you need the security of well-designed restraints. Here are the safety features that safety experts, including the National Highway Traffic Safety Administration, the American Automobile Association, and the Federal Trade Commission, consider most likely to save your life in an accident.

Head restraints. Head restraints cushion your head and neck during a collision. They are required in the front seats of all new passenger vehicles, but some do the job better than others. The best head restraints—usually found on luxury cars—cradle the neck and back of the head and flex during an accident. Make sure the head restraint is positioned directly behind the back of your head, says the Insurance Institute for Highway Safety. Also make sure that an adjustable restraint locks in place exactly where you want it.

Advanced shoulder belts. When a collision occurs, what auto manufacturers call advanced shoulder belts reel in any loose tension that could allow your body to shoot forward against the steering wheel or dashboard. These belts fit more snugly—and they react more quickly during an emergency. The Insurance Institute for Highway Safety reports that they can be found in all 1998 Audi, BMW, Jaguar, Lexus, Mercedes, Saab, Volkswagen, and Volvo models, the 1998 Acura NSX and 3.5 RL; Cadillac Catera and Seville; Chevrolet Prizm and Venture; GM minivans; Honda CR-V; Infiniti Q45; Mitsubishi Diamante; Oldsmobile Silhouette; Pontiac Trans Sport; and all Toyotas except 4Runner and Tacoma.

For a free copy of the Insurance Institute for Highway Safety's pamphlet "Buying a Safer Car," write: Insurance Institute for Highway Safety, 1005 N. Glebe Rd., Suite 800, Arlington, VA 22201.

 Avoid sport utility vehicles.

It's probably no surprise to learn that when a sport utility vehicle (SUV) is involved in a multi-vehicle accident, the driver or passenger of the other smaller vehicle is three times more likely to die. Just looking at the stocky SUVs tells you why: They are heavier, higher from the ground, and more rigid than passenger cars. What may be surprising, however, is that SUVs don't do a lot to protect *their own* drivers in the event of an accident. In fact, they may be more deadly. Keep these facts in mind when you make a decision on whether to buy an SUV.

The major problem with SUVs is they are high riders. When a high-off-the-ground SUV hits a curb or other object, it's likely to flip. Flipping is so common and so deadly that almost one-third of all 1996 passenger car and light truck and van deaths were due to rollover. (SUVs are in the "light truck and van" category.) During single-vehicle accidents, occupants of SUVs have a 46 percent higher death rate because of rollover than those in passenger cars.

When a rollover happens, the driver and passengers are likely to be ejected from the vehicle if they aren't wearing seat belts, or to be injured or even to die. Sixty percent of the time, occupants are thrown through doors or windows. In other cases, the roof collapses, causing head and neck injuries.

Other factors also make SUVs more deadly. They don't have the same stopping distance as passenger cars because their large size requires a longer braking distance. And their rigid truck frames don't absorb the shock of a crash well, says the Insurance Institute for Highway Safety.

Are there any truly safe SUVs? The institute doesn't think so. None of the eight models it tested for crashworthiness rated a "best pick" classification.

 Stay off fast-moving interstates.

Want to make it to 100? Stay away from 65. That is, 65 mph. As states choose to permit speed limits above 55 on their rural interstate highways, you should choose other routes to make sure you reach your destination.

Chances are you already live in a state with new speed limits above 55 mph. The majority of states have upped their speed limits from what had been the nationally mandated 55 mph. Others are in the process of doing so. The result? Additional deaths. By comparison, states that didn't increase the speed limit above 55 mph had decreases in auto fatalities.

The National Highway Traffic Safety Administration estimates that during the time the federal 55 mph limit was in place, up to 30,000 lives were saved.

Although highway fatalities actually decreased in 1996, a total of 41,907 people still died on our roadways. And there was a 10 percent increase in deaths that occurred in the states with the faster-paced roads compared with the year before. To decrease your chance of becoming an accident victim, avoid these faster-paced roads.

■ 70 mph rural interstates in Alabama, Arkansas, California, Florida, Georgia, Kansas, Louisiana, Michigan, Minnesota, Mississippi, Missouri, North Carolina, North Dakota, Tennessee, Texas, Washington, and West Virginia

■ 75 mph rural interstates in Arizona, Colorado, Idaho, Nebraska, Nevada, New Mexico, Oklahoma, South Dakota, Wyoming, and Utah

■ No-limit "reasonable and prudent" speed requirement for interstates in Montana

 ## *Avoid drivers who have been drinking.*

You know they're out there. The newspapers are full of sad stories about how a drunken driver killed a whole family on the way to grandma's house—or how a carload of young people died on the night of their prom. More than 17,000 people were killed in alcohol-related crashes in 1996—almost half of all motor vehicle deaths. And alcohol and speeding go hand in hand. That same year, 42 percent of drivers involved in fatal crashes were not only drunk but also speeding. You can lessen your chances of becoming a fatal statistic if you stay off the road at peak accident hours. Three out of four of the fatal accidents that involved speeding, drunken drivers occurred between the hours of midnight and 3 A.M.

Whenever you travel, watch for the warning signs police officers use to spot drunken drivers. Steer clear of anyone who appears to be doing the following:

■ Turning with a wide radius
■ Straddling the center or lane marker
■ Almost striking an object or vehicle
■ Weaving or swerving
■ Following another vehicle too closely
■ Braking erratically
■ Accelerating or decelerating rapidly

Don't drive drowsy.

Sleepy drivers cause about 4 percent of all fatal crashes each year—and 31 percent of crashes that are fatal to the drivers of commercial trucks. The American Medical Association believes that these numbers are vastly underestimated.

Pull off the road immediately and find a safe place to sleep before continuing your journey if you recognize any of these sleep-deprived signs.

- Your eyes are closing by themselves or going out of focus.
- Your head doesn't stay up.
- You keep yawning.
- Your thoughts are disconnected.
- You forgot what you did during the last few minutes.
- Your driving deteriorates—you drift between lanes or off the road, tailgate, or run red lights or stop signs.

 ## Protect yourself when flying high.

It might seem improbable, but it's possible to survive a plane crash. Follow these tips from safety experts to increase your likelihood of being among the 10 percent who walk away from an air disaster.

✔ **Choose your seating.** Experts consider two areas among the safest places to be seated if a plane crashes. One is right next to an exit door so you can quickly escape. The other is close to the wings—where the plane's stronger structure may protect you.

✔ **Listen to the attendant.** The flight attendant's preflight briefing will help you locate exits, life preservers, and oxygen. Count the rows to the exits in front of you and behind you. This could prove helpful in the event you have to move through a smoky cabin with low visibility.

✔ **Keep heavy items out of the overhead bins.** The last thing you want in an emergency is to be hit by the jar of your Aunt Margaret's boysenberry preserves you've stashed in the overhead bin. If you have something extra heavy, it may be wise to check it at the counter.

✔ **Pick nonstops, if possible.** Most air disasters happen during takeoffs and landings.

✔ **Stay attached.** Keep your seat belt fastened whenever you aren't moving about the cabin. Many injuries occur when passengers are thrown upward and their heads hit the cabin ceiling.

✔ **Wear natural fabrics.** Natural fabrics such as cotton and wool are less likely to ignite in the event of a fire. Synthetic fabrics burn faster and then melt and cling to your body.

✔ **Keep your blood circulating.** Sitting for prolonged periods in a cramped space raises your risk of deep vein thrombosis, a clot that forms in a vein in your leg. The clot can travel to your heart and cause a heart attack, or to your brain and cause a stroke.

You can prevent this from happening by keeping the blood circulating in your legs. On a long flight, walk around the cabin. When seated, flex your leg muscles.

✔ **Use a major airline.** If your plane carries more than 30 passengers, the company is required to meet strict federal safety regulations.

✔ **Choose an airline that equips planes with lifesaving machines.** Several airlines now carry a combination heart monitor and defibrillator—to produce EKGs and shock the heart back into rhythm—on board. Credited with saving the lives of heart attack victims, the devices are available on most American Airlines, Delta Air Lines, Alaska Airlines, and Quantas flights. American is also beefing up its onboard medical supplies to include drugs to treat cardiac arrest, asthma attacks, psychosis, and seizures. Other airlines are expected to follow.

Outdoor Safety

 Protect yourself when participating in sports activities.

The more widely done recreational activities cause the most deaths and injuries, according to the Consumer Product Safety Commission

(CPSC). In-line skating, for example, has caused 25 deaths since 1992, with the number of deaths doubling from 1993 to 1994. And more than 900 people are killed annually in bicycle accidents. In most cases, participants didn't bother to wear the protective gear that may have saved their lives. Here's the commission's 1996 injury count for sports activities, along with ways you can avoid injury and death from the activities you are most likely to enjoy.

Bicycling (nonmountain)	530,274
Mountain biking	27,827
Snow skiing	108,385
In-line skating	102,820
Horseback riding	60,208
Boating	4,589

Bicycling. Sixty percent of all bike accidents involve head injuries, so always don a helmet before hopping on your bike. According to the CPSC, you should wear the helmet flat on the top of your head, tighten the chin strap securely under your chin, and make sure the helmet doesn't block your vision. Another safety precaution for bicyclists: When riding in the street, always ride *with* the traffic.

Skiing. If you're a beginner, take skiing lessons before you hit the slopes. When skiing, keep in control and ski on runs that are within your ability. Maintain a distance of at least 25 feet between yourself and other skiers. Make sure you have appropriate equipment.

In-line skating. Wear protective gear, including a helmet. Don't skate in the streets, where hazards and traffic can cause accidents. And learn how to stop!

Horseback riding. Approximately 30 million Americans climb into the saddle every year, thousands are injured, and some are killed. After all, horses can weigh up to 1,500 pounds, travel as fast as 30 mph, and stand as tall as 6 feet. According to statistics, an equestrian is at risk for a serious accident once every 350 riding hours, with most injuries resulting from a fall off the horse. Deaths usually result from head injuries. Hard shell helmets—securely fastened—should be worn at all times when you are mounted.

Boating. The good news is that U.S. boating fatalities are at an all-time low. The National Association of State Boating Law Administrators says the number of people killed in recreational boating accidents continued to decline in 1996, dropping to a record low of 714. Nonfatal boating accidents also dropped–to 4,589–this even as the number of boat owners and operators continued to grow.

Fatal accidents, however, continue to happen. The primary cause of boating accidents is operator error: inattention, carelessness, and speeding. As many as 90 percent of fatalities occur on boats whose operator had no formal boating instruction, the U.S. Coast Guard calculates. And some 75 percent of victims aren't wearing personal flotation devices. Capsizing due to overloading is also a cause of deaths. Alcohol is a contributing factor in at least half of all boating accidents, the National Safe Boating Council estimates.

To protect yourself from becoming a boating statistic, get boating safety training, available from your local American Red Cross and U.S. Coast Guard; don't drink while operating a boat; don't speed; don't overload your boat; and always wear a flotation device.

 Don't let lightning strike once.

Every year, about 100,000 thunderstorms occur in the United States, complete with nature's spectacular fireworks display: lightning. Almost 100 people are killed by lightning annually when bolts of millions of volts of electricity connect with the ground–an event that occurs about 30 million times a year. And now, researchers believe lightning can kill people without apparently entering or leaving their bodies or without producing visible marks. Electromagnetic discharges from lightning bolts passing close to people without touching them can create a current in the body strong enough to stop the heart cold. To avoid lightning and lightning strikes, follow these precautions from the Centers for Disease Control and Prevention.

✔ **Be aware of when lightning might strike.** Begin to move inside as soon as a storm looks imminent. Lightning can strike even before a drop of rain hits the ground. Nine out of 10 lightning-related deaths happen between May and September–thunderstorm season–when people are more likely to be outdoors. And most deaths occur in the late afternoon or early evening.

✔ **Stay low to the ground.** Lightning is attracted to anything that rises above the landscape, so never seek shelter under a tree or under an open structure such as an observation tower. If lightning zaps a tree or structure, the electricity is conducted downward—and into any bystander. If you're in an open field, crouch down or look for a low-lying ditch or ravine.

✔ **Avoid heavy metal.** Stay away from golf clubs and carts, umbrellas, and tools. Metal fences are also dangerous lightning magnets. If you are on a bike or tractor, get off and move several feet away.

✔ **Stay away from electrical conductors inside your house.** For the best protection, install lightning rods on your roof. When lightning hits a house without lightning rods, the current can travel through telephone wires or plumbing. During thunderstorms, avoid the telephone, plumbing, fireplaces, windows, and electronic appliances (which should be turned off).

✔ **Stash that cellular phone.** Cellular phones are lightning attractors. Don't use yours during a thunderstorm if you are near any open areas outside or are near a window.

 ## Protect yourself against disease-carrying ticks.

Ticks can do much more than set you scratching. More than 10,000 cases of Lyme disease were reported in 1997. The bacterial infection is carried by deer ticks, which feed on deer and then hang out on low vegetation until passersby brush up against them. The ticks then can burrow into your skin to transmit an infection of the bacterium *Borrelia burgdorferi*, which can cause rash, flulike symptoms, and, rarely, neurological and heart problems. Arthritis may also develop, especially in the knees.

Lyme disease has been reported in nearly all states, although most cases are concentrated in the coastal Northeast, mid-Atlantic states, Wisconsin and Minnesota, and northern California. (In California, the culprit is the western black-legged tick.) In addition, another tick-carried disease, Rocky Mountain spotted fever, is found in all states, especially along the Atlantic seaboard. This disease can lead to pneumonia, heart and brain damage–and sometimes death. And ehrlichiosis, which resembles Rocky Mountain spotted fever but is carried by the brown dog tick, is also found everywhere. It causes high fever and flulike illness, which is often fatal if left untreated. Here's how to prevent, recognize, and treat tick-generated diseases if you live in an area where they occur.

✔ **Be a smart dresser.** When walking in wooded areas where deer are likely to be present, wear long-sleeved shirts tucked into long pants. Tuck the pants legs into hiking boots or socks. Ticks like the scalp, so wear a hat. Light-colored clothing makes the ticks easier to find.

✔ **Use insect repellents carefully.** Repellents with DEET in them are very effective at keeping ticks and most other insects at bay. For a few people, however, such repellents may cause problems. Adverse reactions have been reported in adults, but infants and children are particularly at risk when small amounts of the chemical enter the skin and cause allergic reactions such as breathing difficulties or seizures. Choose insecticides with low DEET concentrations. Spray them on clothing and shoes to help repel ticks. Don't keep reapplying the repellent as you hike. And never spray on broken skin.

✔ **Check yourself out.** After a hike in the woods or a Saturday working in the garden, do a thorough skin check. Make sure you do this soon after possible tick exposure–it takes 24 to 48 hours for ticks to transmit disease. With the help of a partner, don't forget to examine your scalp.

✔ **Remove the tick.** Never use your fingers, which can become infected. Instead, take tweezers and gently pull, getting as close to the skin as possible. This may make the tick release its grip on your skin. Try to avoid twisting the tick's head or otherwise crushing the tick because either action may allow the insect to release its bacteria into your skin. After the tick is removed, gently wash the area of the bite with soap and water and apply an antiseptic.

✔ **Hold on to the tick.** Save the tick in a glass jar with alcohol in case you develop any symptoms of Lyme disease. (The specimen can help your doctor make a definitive diagnosis.) You should also make a note of the geographic area you were in when you think you were bitten.

✔ **Don't treat Lyme before it's time.** A study reported in the *Journal of the American Medical Association* pointed out that physicians often diagnose and treat Lyme disease when it doesn't exist. There is no reliable test for the bacterium that causes Lyme disease, so doctors must use symptoms to diagnose the condition. About three-quarters of those infected have a large red spot, which expands to about 6 inches. This is commonly called the "bull's eye" rash. Flulike symptoms then may follow. Antibiotic treatment at any stage is effective, but early treatment helps prevent complications. A laboratory test to analyze your levels of antibodies to the bacterium may help decide whether antibiotics are necessary.

 ## Don't drink from mountain streams or lakes.

What could be more picturesque than a bubbling stream rushing down the hillside? And you found it just in time to take a drink and refill your canteen. . . . Screw that lid back on; the water may be dangerous to your health.

Lakes and streams that are downhill from animal-raising farms or even campsites may be contaminated with fecal bacteria or with disease-causing giardiasis parasites. The parasites, which normally are found at the silty bottoms of slow streams, can be dispersed throughout the water in fast-flowing streams. If ingested, the parasites can cause nausea, abdominal pain, and diarrhea or prevent nutrients from being adequately absorbed from food.

If you're drinking water outdoors, carry your own or boil local sources for three minutes. Adding iodine tablets to the water also kills bacteria.

4 Lifestyle Choices

Most people who live longer have an important thing in common: They don't engage in behavior that could jeopardize their health.

Your lifestyle is the one determining factor of health and longevity over which you have total control. In this chapter, we look at lifestyle choices you can make to promote good health and add years to your life.

Exercise

 Exercise away your risk of disease.

Medical studies overwhelmingly confirm that exercise can lower the risk of life-threatening diseases. A 1995 study of 17,000 Harvard University alumni, for example, found that men who exercised vigorously enough to burn at least 1,500 calories a week had a 25 percent lower mortality rate than men who didn't exercise. In another study, reported in the *Journal of the American Medical Association*, out of 40,000 postmenopausal women studied for seven years, those who exercised regularly were 20 percent less likely to die during the period than their sedentary counterparts.

Here are the major diseases that exercise helps exorcise.

Heart disease and stroke. The studies confirm it time and again: If you exercise regularly, your risk of heart attack is reduced – to as much as half that of a sedentary person, according to a report in the *New England Journal of Medicine*. But if you don't exercise, your risk of heart disease is comparable to that of someone who smokes or has blood pressure or high cholesterol, the Centers for Disease Control and Prevention points out. Sedentary people are 80 percent more likely to develop heart disease than active people, according to the MacArthur Foundation Study on Successful Aging.

Exercise also lowers your likelihood of a life-threatening stroke. One study, published in the *Annals of Internal Medicine*, showed that the risk of fatal stroke was 60 percent lower in Dutch men who exercised than in Dutch men who were sedentary. And moderate exercise for at least an hour five times a week can reduce stroke risk by up to 50 percent, according to a 1998 study reported in the journal *Stroke*.

Regular physical activity changes the way the body handles free radicals, oxygen-scavenging molecules that allow low-density lipoprotein (LDL, the "bad" cholesterol) to build up dangerous plaque in arteries. Regular aerobic exercise increases enzymes that neutralize the free radicals. Furthermore, exercise affects the endothelium, the lining of the blood vessels. When you exercise, the endothelium sends chemical signals that cause your blood vessels to dilate. Blood vessels that dilate frequently are more flexible and less likely to have pockets where plaque can form.

High blood pressure. According to the American College of Sports Medicine, exercise can reduce moderately high blood pressure—both systolic and diastolic—by at least 10 mm Hg.

Breast cancer. Several studies show that exercise reduces the risk of breast cancer. Researchers in Norway, for example, monitored the exercise habits of more than 25,000 women and found that those who exercised at least four hours a week had a 37 percent lower risk of developing breast cancer than those who were sedentary. Another study, from the University of Southern California, found a reduction of 40 percent with just over three and one-half hours a week of exercise. Although it's not known for sure why exercise may reduce breast cancer risk, it's believed to be related to the fact that exercise lowers levels of estrogen in the body.

Colon cancer. There's evidence that physical activity protects against colon cancer, which is more prevalent in overweight individuals. In one study, reported in the *Journal of the National Cancer Institute*, women who exercised the most had half the risk of colon cancer as women who exercised the least. Men are equally protected. A Harvard University study showed that men who walked just a few hours a week reduced their colon cancer risk by 30 percent.

Infectious diseases. Preliminary studies have shown that regular exercise exerts a positive influence on the immune system. Exercise helps prevent minor infectious illnesses such as colds and flu and has been shown to slow the progression of AIDS. Exercise increases the immune system's natural killer cells and the T cells that provoke the immune response. Exercise also raises the body's levels of endogenous pyrogen, a fever-causing protein, which results in a higher body temperature that slows down viruses and bacteria, thus making them easier targets for the immune system. In addition, exercise speeds up metabolism, possibly flushing carcinogens out of the body.

Exercise may also slow the natural decline of the immune system that comes with age. A study reported in *Sports Medicine Digest* showed that endurance training such as running increased the immune system function of Japanese men. The exercise slowed down age-related decline in both T cell function and the production of interleukin-2, a protein that facilitates the production of T cells.

Diabetes. Exercise can help reduce the risk of diabetes and help control it if it does develop. During exercise, muscles rapidly use their own stores of glycogen and triglycerides, as well as fatty acids derived from the breakdown of fatty tissue triglycerides and glucose released from the liver. In patients with type 2 diabetes, exercise may improve insulin sensitivity and reduce elevated blood glucose levels. In addition, exercise helps delay or stop cardiovascular disease, the leading killer of people with diabetes. And for people who are diagnosed with type 2 diabetes, exercise combined with proper diet often eliminates the need for insulin.

Osteoporosis. Osteoporosis, the brittle bone disease, can lead to life-threatening hip fractures, particularly in postmenopausal women. Studies show that weight-bearing exercise—lifting weights, walking or jogging, and dancing, to name some prominent examples—increases bone mass and prevents fractures. As little as one hour a week reduces the risk of hip fractures, reports a study in the *Annals of Internal*

Medicine. Researchers monitored more than 9,700 women ages 65 and older for seven years and found that those women who were moderately to vigorously active were up to 42 percent less likely to have hip and vertebral fractures than their inactive counterparts.

 ## Get 30 *minutes of exercise daily.*

The Surgeon General recommends that every adult in America accumulate 30 minutes or more of moderate-intensity physical activity on most, preferably all, days of the week. But according to the Centers for Disease Control and Prevention (CDC), only about half of Americans get the daily exercise they need to be healthy.

Exercise often conjures up the image of glistening bodies working off that last pucker of cellulite in an expensive gym or of hikers with a pack the size of Mt. Everest making for that next ridge. But exercise can be as close as your own backyard or living room. Walking, gardening, raking leaves, taking the stairs, doing housework, and playing with the kids are considered exercise and can count toward your daily total, as can any regular sports activity, such as tennis, aerobics, golf, or cycling.

If you already have at least 30 minutes of exercise in your daily schedule, the CDC recommends that you pick up the pace to derive even more health benefits.

 ## Get your exercise in short sessions.

If you find it difficult to get to a gym regularly or even take 30 minutes for a run around the park, try regular 10-minute sessions at home. Cumulatively, they are as valuable as a longer session of aerobic exercise, research shows.

During a four-month study at the University of Pittsburgh School of Medicine, obese women were asked to limit calories to fewer than 1,500 and exercise five times weekly. The women were assigned one of three exercise regimens: a single, 40-minute session of any exercise, 10 minutes of any exercise four times daily, and 10 minutes four times daily on a home treadmill. The shorter sessions proved more beneficial because those who exercised in their homes were most likely to stick with the routine; they were also most successful at losing their extra pounds.

Exercise doesn't just have to be jogging, biking, and swimming. You can also make lifestyle changes to get exercise in short, but important, spurts. Love your remote control? Stash it away and get up to change TV channels. Park your car at a distance from the mall entrance when you go shopping or bike to a local shop. Take the stairs whenever possible. And don't use your kids as gofers—get whatever you need yourself.

 ## Walk your way to longevity.

It's easy on the body, it's enjoyable, it's inexpensive, and you can do it with friends. But the best thing about walking on a regular basis is that it can increase your chances of living longer.

Here's what researchers have found out about the longevity benefits of walking.

■ Researchers who analyzed the health and exercise patterns of nonsmokers taking part in the Honolulu Heart Program found that the more the study participants walked, the less likely they were to die of cardiovascular diseases and cancer. Nonsmoking study participants who walked more than two miles a day had the lowest mortality rate.

■ In what they called the first study to separate the effects of heredity and exercise on longevity, researchers tracked 8,000 sets of twins for 19 years. The study, reported in the *Journal of the American Medical Association*, found that twins who took moderate walks were one-third less likely to die during the period than their more sedentary womb mates. The more vigorous their walks, the longer they survived. Those who walked briskly or jogged for at least 30 minutes six times monthly were 44 percent less likely to die during the study period than those who didn't exercise.

■ The benefits of beginning a walking program may be long lasting. Researchers from the University of Minnesota and the University of Pittsburgh interviewed a group of women who a decade earlier had volunteered for a study to evaluate walking's health benefits. Those who had been encouraged to walk for daily exercise had continued to do so, and their health was better than that of those who had not been encouraged to walk. They experienced fewer hospitalizations, surgeries, and falls, and their rate of heart disease was a low 2.4 percent compared with the sedentary group's 12.9 percent rate.

YOUR TARGET HEART RATE ZONE

To get health benefits from aerobic activity, exercise at a level that will raise your heart rate to your target zone. Count the number of pulse beats at your wrist for 15 seconds, then multiply by four to get the beats per minute. Your target heart rate zone is 50 to 75 percent of your maximum heart rate (the fastest your heart can beat). If your heart is beating faster, you are exercising too hard and should slow down.

To find your target zone, look for the category closest to your age in the chart below.

Age (Years)	Target Heart Rate Zone (50-75 percent)	Average Maximum Heart Rate (100 percent)
20	100–150	200
25	98–146	195
30	95–142	190
35	93–138	185
40	90–135	180
45	88–131	175
50	85–127	170
55	83–123	165
60	80–120	160
65	78–116	155
70	75–113	150

Source: National Institutes of Health.

Behavioral Changes

 Floss and brush to stay healthy.

Some 75 percent of the over-55 population has some form of periodontal (gum) disease. And studies are now linking gum disease to an increased risk of heart disease and stroke. Those who have their teeth cleaned annually are five times less likely to have strokes than those who have less frequent cleanings, according to a University of Michigan School of Dentistry study.

The relationship between gum disease and heart disease and stroke is not as fanciful as you might first think. Several mechanisms may be involved. When bacteria build up on the teeth, plaque is formed. The most common bacterium in dental plaque is *Streptococcus sanguis*, which has been shown to foster blood clots. The pockets created when unhealthy gums pull away from the teeth are breeding grounds for bacteria. Researchers believe that when bacteria are not controlled by proper dental hygiene, they may trigger blood clots in the arteries, possibly due to the inflammation associated with infection. If the arteries are already clogged with atherosclerotic plaque, a heart attack or stroke may be the fatal result.

To keep your teeth and your body healthy, spend at least three minutes nightly flossing and brushing.

 Use sunscreen.

You've heard the warnings about skin cancer: One million people in the United States are diagnosed with it every year, according to the American Cancer Society (ACS). This makes skin cancer the most common cancer in America. And the incidence of the most deadly form of skin cancer, melanoma, has increased about 4 percent annually since 1973. Melanoma accounts for less than 5 percent of skin cancer cases but causes about 79 percent of skin cancer deaths, the ACS reports. In 1998, an estimated 41,600 new cases were diagnosed, with an estimated 7,300 deaths. Those at highest risk are people who sunburn easily, have red or blond hair, or have fair skin.

Fortunately, you can reduce your risk of skin cancer by taking these precautions.

✔ *Always wear sunscreen.* Ninety percent of sun exposure comes during ordinary activities. Even on cloudy days, ultraviolet (UV) exposure is reduced only by 20 percent.

✔ *Use the right kind of sunscreen.* According to the American Academy of Dermatology, you should use sunscreen with an SPF (sun protection factor) of at least 15. At least 15 minutes before you go out, apply the sunscreen (or a sunblock to completely block the rays) to all exposed areas of the skin, including the backs of the knees, lips, eyelids (be careful not to get it in your eyes), ears, feet, and bare scalp. If you're going to be swimming, use a waterproof sunblock.

✔ *Avoid tanning beds.* Tanning salons use UVA radiation, which is less likely to burn than the shorter-wave UVB rays. But UVA rays penetrate more deeply into the skin, inhibiting immune reactions and making skin cancer more likely. Furthermore, the booths emit two to three times more UVA than the sun.

 Prevent sexually transmitted diseases.

More than 12 million Americans are infected with sexually transmitted diseases (STDs) annually—many unknowingly because the symptoms often don't appear for years. According to the Centers for Disease Control and Prevention, up to 40 percent of the sexually active adult population has some form of STD. While most of the more than 20 STDs are only painful and unpleasant, some are deadly. Here are the ones that can shorten your life span.

HIV (human immunodeficiency virus). HIV causes AIDS, the fifth leading cause of death in people between the ages of 25 and 44 in the United States. AIDS was responsible for 16,685 deaths in 1997, and although the death rate is at its lowest level since 1987, the number of new infections has held steady at about 40,000 annually. AIDS, an incurable disease, attacks the body's immune system, leaving it susceptible to fatal infections and cancers. HIV is spread through contact with infected body fluids, including semen and blood. Initial symptoms include fever, rash, and swollen lymph nodes. A blood test can detect the presence of the HIV antibodies.

Human papillomavirus (HPV). As many as 40 percent of college women may be infected with this virus, which causes genital warts. HPV is symptomless in about three-fourths of those infected, but it is a major contributor to cervical cancer in women. It may also contribute to penile cancer in men. The warts may be removed surgically or chemically, but the virus remains latent. Infected women should have annual Pap smears to screen for cervical cancer.

Hepatitis B. Hepatitis B is a liver infection 100 times more infectious than HIV. Each year, about 300,000 Americans get hepatitis B, which leads to permanent liver disease or cancer of the liver in about 10 percent of those infected. Not a strictly sexually transmitted disease, hepatitis B is spread through contact with infected body fluids, including semen, saliva, and blood. Health care workers and others at risk for the virus can be immunized. Symptoms include poor appetite, nausea, vomiting, fever, and joint pains. Symptoms and a blood test of liver functions are used to diagnose infection with the virus.

Syphilis. Syphilis is a bacterial disease that can lead to heart and brain damage and death if left untreated. Contracted primarily through sexual intercourse, its symptoms include a painless sore that appears on the genitals, mouth, or elsewhere up to three months after infection. A fever, rash, and flulike symptoms may appear about six weeks after the initial symptoms. A blood test can indicate presence of the bacterium, but results may not be accurate for up to 12 weeks after infection. Penicillin is used to treat all stages of the disease and usually effects a cure.

Gonorrhea. This bacterial infection, which affects an estimated 2 million people each year, may not have noticeable symptoms. Gonorrhea can be treated and cured with antibiotics. Left untreated, however, it can lead to complications, including ectopic pregnancy, which is potentially fatal to the pregnant woman. A doctor takes a sample of discharge from the penis or a cervical smear and then identifies the gonococcus bacterium under a microscope.

To make sure you don't become infected with these potentially fatal conditions, take these steps.

✔ **Use latex condoms whether you are using other birth control methods or not.** Use condoms in conjunction with a jelly, cream, or foam that contains nonoxynol-9. Although it may help reduce the spread of other STDs, nonoxynol-9 is no longer thought to prevent the transmission of HIV. And condoms with the spermicide have not been found to be more effective at preventing STDs than regular condoms, according to a study by researchers at Family Health International in Durham, North Carolina.

✔ **Don't share needles, syringes, or instruments used in ear-piercing, tattooing, or hair removal.** Some STDs, such as HIV, hepatitis B, and syphilis, can also be spread through the exchange of blood and other body fluids. Toothbrushes can also transmit hepatitis B, so reserve yours for yourself.

✔ **If you are sexually active—especially with a new partner or multiple partners—have regular checkups for STDs.** These tests can be done during a routine visit to the doctor's office.

✔ **Abstain from sex or participate only in a long-term monogamous relationship with an uninfected partner.** In addition, young people should delay having sexual relations as long as possible, the National Institutes of Health counsels. The younger people are when having sex for the first time, the more susceptible they become to developing STDs. The risk of acquiring an STD also increases with the number of partners over a lifetime.

 Stop smoking.

One in five of all deaths in the United States is due to cigarette smoking. Up to age 65, smokers who smoke at least a pack a day—20 cigarettes or more—have double the death rate of nonsmokers. The biggest risks to longevity are from cancers of the lungs, throat, and mouth. Pack-a-day cigarette smokers are 14 times more likely to die of these diseases. Esophageal and bladder cancers are also found at higher rates in smokers. And women who smoke are at higher risk for cervical cancer. Smoking also contributes to heart disease—at least 200,000 smokers and up to 40,000 nonsmokers who have regularly been exposed to tobacco smoke die of heart disease each year.

The good news is that many of these health risks can be reversed when you stop smoking. In fact, your lungs begin to clear themselves from unhealthy toxins in as few as 20 minutes after you have had your last puff. After 10 years, the risk of lung cancer is about the same as that of a nonsmoker's. Heart attack risk is cut in half in the first year after quitting.

Put out your cigar too. Despite their growing popularity (use of the expensive premium variety has increased by 250 percent since 1993), cigars have the same potential as cigarettes to cause heart disease and cancer, according to Daniel Sterman, M.D., of the University of Pennsylvania Medical Center. Regular cigar smokers have double the risk of dying from all types of cancer. They also have a higher risk of dangerous circulatory problems caused by high blood pressure and cardiomyopathy (deterioration of the lower pumping chambers of the heart). Cigar smokers are also at risk for oral cancer and cancer of the larynx. If they inhale, they have the same risk of lung cancer as cigarette smokers do.

To stop smoking, heed these prequitting tips from the National Cancer Institute and select one or more smoking cessation methods from the chart that follows.

✔ *Switch to a brand you find distasteful.*

✔ *Cut down on the number of cigarettes you smoke.* Smoke only half of each cigarette, postpone your first cigarette by an hour, and decide beforehand how many cigarettes to smoke daily.

✔ *Don't empty your ashtrays.* This will remind you how many cigarettes you've smoked.

✔ *Put your cigarettes in a different pocket or location to break the automatic reach.*

✔ *Buy cigarettes only one pack at a time.*

✔ *Don't carry cigarettes with you.*

Smoking Cessation Methods

THERAPY	HOW IT WORKS	EFFECTIVENESS
Zyban (bupropion) Zyban is a nonnicotine drug approved for smoking cessation.	Zyban is an antidepressant that reduces the urge to smoke and alleviates some of the withdrawal symptoms such as anxiety, irritability, and depression that accompany the removal of nicotine from your body.	One study has shown that that more than half of those who used Zyban with a nicotine patch were able to stop smoking.
Nicotine The addictive substance in cigarettes and cigars can also be used as a smoking cessation treatment.	Available in patch, gum, or nasal spray form, nicotine smoking cessation treatments help smokers gradually withdraw from the nicotine in cigarettes and cigars.	Nicotine smoking cessation treatments are only adjuncts to quitting. They help reduce physical craving while they are being used, but they cannot be used indefinitely.
Behavior modification The highest quitting success rates are among those who benefit from behavior modification techniques learned as part of a support group.	In four to seven sessions, you learn to identify your smoking triggers, how to cope with withdrawal, what to substitute for cigarettes, how to cope with weight gain, and how to remain a nonsmoker.	Works well in conjunction with medications or with therapies such as acupuncture, hypnosis, and biofeedback.

Drink only in moderation, if at all.

Although numerous studies have found that light-to-moderate alcohol consumption reduces the risk of heart disease and light consumption reduces the risk of ischemic stroke, alcohol can also increase the risk of disease and injury. Even light-to-moderate alcohol consumption has been linked in some studies to an increased risk of cirrhosis, hemorrhagic stroke, breast cancer, and injuries. Heavier consumption is known to increase the risk of mouth, throat, colon, and liver cancers, as well as heart disease and ischemic stroke.

Here's a sampling of the research.

Heart disease. A nine-year study of nearly half a million men and women, reported in a 1997 issue of the *New England Journal of Medicine*, found that alcohol's beneficial effects are tied to a person's age, heart condition, and alcohol intake. Overall mortality was 20 percent lower in study participants who drank one alcoholic beverage a day than in nondrinkers. Above one drink, however, death rates increased. Death rates for drinkers ages 60 to 79 with heart disease remained significantly lower than those of nondrinkers, even in those who reported drinking four or more drinks a day, but death rates for younger, healthy participants who reported drinking four or more drinks a day were significantly higher than those of nondrinkers.

Stroke. In a 1998 study, Austrian researchers examined the effects of alcohol consumption on the development of atherosclerosis in the carotid arteries, the arteries that supply blood to the brain. Blockage of these arteries can lead to stroke. They found that men and women who drank less than 50 grams of alcohol per day (comparable to two glasses of beer or wine) had a lower risk of carotid atherosclerosis than heavy drinkers and nondrinkers. Heavy drinkers, on the other hand, (those who drank 100 grams or more per day) had a risk greater than that of heavy smokers.

Breast cancer. A large Harvard University study made headlines in 1998 for finding that even light-to-moderate drinking substantially raises a woman's risk of breast cancer. The study, reported the *Journal of the American Medical Association*, found that women who drank two to five alcoholic drinks daily increased their risk of developing invasive breast cancer by 41 percent. Each daily drink was associated with an approximate 9 percent increase in risk.

If you drink, limit your daily alcohol intake. The Dietary Guidelines for Americans recommend that women drink no more than one drink a day and men drink no more than two drinks a day. A drink is 12 ounces of beer, 5 ounces of wine, or 1½ ounces of 80-proof liquor.

 ## Use self-efficacy techniques to modify unhealthy behavior.

You rolled off the couch and started to take a daily walk to help lower your high blood pressure. Or you cut out trips to the ice cream shop and lost five pounds in time for your high school reunion. How did you make these changes? You instinctively used a form of behavior modification called self-efficacy. You changed your behavior to serve personal needs that range from avoiding illness to improving your body image. But don't stop now. You can use self-efficacy to change your behavior to decrease other risky behaviors.

✔ **Be specific.** Instead of vowing to eat a healthy diet, for example, set up a detailed diet plan that includes no more than the U.S. Department of Agriculture's recommended amounts for problem areas such as fats and sweets. In addition, plan your meals, including those you eat out.

✔ **Handle your hot spots.** Addicted to Ben & Jerry's Chubby Hubby? Keep it out of the freezer. Instead of buying prepackaged ice cream, limit yourself to a single scoop serving at your favorite ice cream shop once or twice a month.

✔ **Practice, practice, practice.** Regularly practice your new behavior. Each time you do, you reinforce behavioral change. If you backtrack, don't lose heart. Just continue the new behavior at the next opportunity.

✔ **Revel in rewards.** When your new behavior takes hold, reward yourself. A day at the office when you've controlled stress levels calls for a new CD or a relaxing night with the latest best-seller.

5 ∎ Between Mind and Body

For thousands of years, people thought the human soul resided in the heart. Then modern medicine brought the knowledge that the heart is a complicated system of muscles and valves that function as a pump. Suddenly, it was out with the soul, in with artificial valves and transplants–not to mention angioplasties, bypass surgeries, and a pharmacopoeia of medications. Yet now, medical science has come to know that the mind and soul are as crucial to health and longevity as the heart and other organs. Overall, research shows that people who are connected–with the outside world, family, friends, community of faith–live longer.

Studies also show that the body's cardiovascular and immune systems benefit greatly from people's social connections, as well as their mental well-being. People who keep their minds active and learn to manage the stress in their lives generally experience better health.

Social Connections

 Be *spiritual.*

There is a positive relationship between high levels of faith and higher immune system function and lower incidence of heart disease. According to research, religious affiliation, age, and gender don't make a difference. The connection between better health and spirituality has been made in these studies.

■ When 91,000 Maryland residents were studied, researchers found that those who attended church weekly were half as likely to die of coronary heart disease and emphysema as nonchurchgoers.

■ Older North Carolinians who attended church at least once a week had lower blood pressure readings than did those who went less frequently or not at all, a Duke University study showed. The likelihood of having a diastolic blood pressure of 90 mm Hg or higher was cut by 40 percent when people attended church weekly or studied the Bible daily. (High diastolic readings are associated with heart attacks and strokes.) The study also found that people who regularly tuned in to radio religious programming had higher blood pressure than churchgoers, indicating that the healthy benefits came from the old-fashioned form of church attendance.

■ People with breast cancer, heart disease, or other life-threatening diseases who found comfort in religion were more likely to be alive six months down the road, another Duke University study found.

■ A study of Catholic nuns found that their blood pressure didn't rise as they became older, which is commonly the case as people age. Furthermore, a study of people living in religious kibbutzim and secular kibbutzim in Israel found that the members of religious kibbutzim lived longer than those living in secular kibbutzim.

■ Depressed patients who were hospitalized at Duke University Hospital for conditions such as heart disease and stroke and who scored high on a scale that measured religious commitment recovered faster from their depression.

 Make companionship a priority.

In a study of heart attack patients, published in the *Annals of Internal Medicine*, more than half of those who died within six months of their heart attack had reported at the beginning of the study that they had "no one" to turn to for love or comfort. In contrast, none of the study participants who were socially involved and deeply religious died in the six months following their heart attack.

Studies have shown that older women with close relationships have lower blood pressure–often comparable to that of much younger people. Other research indicates that there may be such as thing as a broken heart: Married people have lower rates of heart attack than widowed or divorced people, and individuals who have just lost a loved one have increased rates of death, most frequently from heart disease.

People with close relationships are three to five times less likely to die prematurely, according to a University of Michigan study. In fact, social isolation is now believed to be a heart disease risk factor, and one perhaps as dangerous as smoking, being overweight, or having high blood pressure, according to Robert Kahn, Ph.D., a member of the MacArthur Foundation Research Network on Successful Aging.

A social support system is one of the most effective ways to reduce the effects of stress on the immune system. An Ohio State

ARE YOU CONNECTED?

Use these questions, based on work by psychologist Sheldon Cohen, Ph.D., to determine if you are socially connected.

■ Do you have someone you can call if you need advice about a personal matter?

■ If you need some physical help–moving furniture or getting a ride somewhere–is there someone you could call?

■ Would anyone take care of your house when you're away on vacation?

■ Would anyone throw a surprise birthday party for you?

■ Do others often ask for your advice or take you into their confidence?

If you answered "no" to one or more of these indicators, it may be time to get out and get connected. Churches and synagogues are good places to meet people who will pinch in when there is a problem. If you are estranged from your family, make a phone call and build some bridges. In addition, cultivate a neighborly friendship with those living close by.

University study found that caregivers of sick spouses had lower levels of stress hormones when they had support from family or friends. In another study, conducted at the Stanford University School of Medicine, people with advanced-stage cancer who attended group therapy doubled clinical expectations for the time left before their cancer-related deaths.

Those who do something for others are also healthier. In a study of people who helped out the Big Brothers/Big Sisters program, those who volunteered weekly were 10 times more likely to report good health.

Mental Wellness

 Identify with being well.

Studies across a wide range of illnesses show that patients who expect to get well often do so, regardless of treatment. This phenomenon is known as the placebo effect. The mind takes over to promote healing. Herbert Benson, M.D., president of the Mind/Body Medical Institute at Beth Israel Deaconess Medical Center in Boston, has another name for this phenomenon: remembered wellness. According to Benson, positive beliefs activate certain patterns in the brain that are associated with wellness.

In one study, for example, patients with physical complaints but no identifiable diseases were told either that no serious diseases had been found and that they soon would be well or that the causes of their ailments were unclear. Two weeks later, 64 percent of the first group had recovered compared with only 39 percent of the second. So whenever you are ill, let your mind focus on healthiness and you'll be more likely to recover and live longer.

 Exercise your mind.

As you get older, certain mental functioning skills decline, especially after age 80. Spacial orientation and inductive reasoning—in which you recognize patterns in order to predict what comes next–decline. You tend to take longer to make decisions, and your memory usually isn't as sharp. On the other hand, vocabulary and math skills actually improve with age, and reasoning ability stays the same, the Baltimore Longitudinal Study of Aging reports.

Here's what experts say will help keep your mind alert.

✔ *Seek stimulating companionship.* The reasoning abilities of spouses become more similar over time, according to *Nutrition Action Newsletter.* Typically, a lower-functioning spouse will move toward the higher-functioning spouse. If you don't have a mate or feel you are the higher-functioning person in the relationship, spend time with other family members or friends who are more stimulating.

✔ *Take classes.* Studies show that the more education you have, the more likely you are to retain your mental functioning. Education appears to increase the number and strength of synapses, the connections between brain cells. A Columbia University study showed that people with less than an eighth-grade education had twice the risk of Alzheimer's disease as those who continued their education. Take courses at local community colleges or night schools. Being willing to change your thinking also keeps the brain fresh.

✔ *Take up a hobby that requires some mental agility.* Collecting antiques, coins, or stamps, doing genealogical research, bird-watching–these all require an expanding knowledge base.

✔ *Play games.* Chess, of course, is the mind-bender of all time, but any games that require reasoning will add to mental alertness as you age. Get friends or family together for regular nights of Scrabble, Cribbage, or card games. Crossword puzzles are also good.

✔ *Avoid stress.* High levels of stress hormones disrupt both short- and long-term memory. Glucocorticoid, a hormone produced by stress, is believed to destroy brain cells.

✔ *Participate in physical exercise.* Active exercise improves blood flow to the brain.

✔ *Seek out new experiences.* Travel, new acquaintances, volunteerism–all contribute to increased connections in the brain.

✔ **Work hard.** Researchers at the MacArthur Foundation Research Network on Successful Aging found that people in their 70s who worked strenuously at any activity were less likely to lose their mental sharpness.

 Enhance your mind with vitamins.

Studies now show that certain vitamins can increase your mental function.

Vitamin B₁₂. An untreated deficiency of this vitamin–from which an estimated 7 to 15 percent of older Americans suffer–can result in irreversible memory loss. If you are over 65 and have some memory loss, talk to your doctor. The Recommended Dietary Allowance (RDA) of vitamin B₁₂ is 2.4 micrograms daily, but Michael Freedman, director of geriatrics at New York University Medical Center, suggests 25 micrograms daily to correct deficiencies. Good food sources of vitamin B₁₂ are meats and fish, particularly salmon.

Vitamin E. A known antioxidant, vitamin E may help prevent cognitive loss. High doses of vitamin E have been shown to slow the progression of Alzheimer's disease, and the American Psychiatric Association includes the vitamin, in doses between 200 and 800 I.U. per day, in its latest treatment guidelines for Alzheimer's disease. The RDA is 15 I.U., or 10 milligrams, for men and 12 I.U., or 8 milligrams, for women. Food sources include wheat germ, vegetable oils, whole grain cereals, eggs, nuts, and seeds.

Folic acid. Low levels of folic acid may be associated with mental decline. The National Academy of Sciences' Food and Nutrition Board, which establishes the RDAs, recently raised the RDA of folic acid to 400 micrograms. Folic acid is found in leafy greens, wheat germ, beans, whole grains, broccoli, and citrus fruit.

 Recognize the symptoms of depression.

Depression can affect not only your mood but also your physical health. Johns Hopkins University School of Medicine researchers found that people who were diagnosed with clinical depression had twice the risk of developing heart disease as people not diagnosed with the condition. Another study, reported in the *American Journal of Cardiology*, found that people with depression and heart disease had a risk of dying from a heart attack up to 84 percent greater than people who weren't depressed.

Occasional dark thoughts are normal and unlikely to affect your health. But if you have the symptoms that follow, you may be among the 10 to 15 percent of the U.S. population who suffers from clinical depression at some time in their lives.

- A persistent sad, anxious or empty feeling
- Loss of interest in activities, including sex
- Restlessness, irritability, or excessive crying
- Feelings of worthlessness, guilt, helplessness, or pessimism
- Sleeping too much or too little
- Eating too much or too little
- Decreased energy
- Difficulty remembering, concentrating, or making decisions
- Thoughts of suicide

According to the National Institute on Aging, if you have at least five of these symptoms of depression for at least two weeks, a physician should evaluate you. The next step would be treatment by a mental health professional.

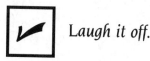 *Laugh it off.*

Laughter is an instant mood elevator. When you laugh, your circulation and digestion improve and your blood pressure drops. Even a simple smile increases blood flow to the brain and releases endorphins, painkilling hormones that make you feel good. Levels of heart-attacking stress hormones drop, decreasing your risk of stroke and heart attack. Further, a fun-loving, humorous personality attracts friends–another proven way to extend your life.

Humor also works in several ways to help your immune system function. For example, humorous people are more likely to use laughter to manage stressful situations. People who use humor to cope with stress have higher infection-fighting immunoglobulin A levels than those who don't, according to researchers at the University of Western Ontario. Another study showed that immunoglobulin A levels increase when people watch a humor video.

 Be an optimist.

If your cup is usually half full rather than half empty, you may be increasing your longevity.

Researchers believe a positive attitude may reverse the unhealthy effects of stressful events, which can negatively affect our immune system. A study published in the *Journal of Personality and Social Psychology*, for example, found that law students who were optimistic were more likely to have healthier immune systems—despite their grueling study schedules. Their immune system's T cells and natural killer cells—specialized cells that help the immune system target and fight harmful invaders such as bacteria and viruses—increased. And HIV-positive men who thought their condition could be controlled experienced an increase in T cells and lived nine months longer than HIV-positive men who were more pessimistic, according to a study conducted at London's Chelsea and Westminster Hospital.

Another study, reported in the journal *Psychological Science*, found that pessimism is a risk factor for early death, especially among men. Pessimists were defined as people who blame themselves when something goes wrong and who feel that one big mistake can ruin a life. They expect bad things to happen to them and don't go out of their way to avoid them. Not surprisingly, pessimists in this study were more likely to die as a result of accidents, violence, and suicide.

If you fit into the pessimist mold, you can change. One way is to seek out cognitive therapy, which helps people identify and change negative thoughts that regularly occur. Another important thing to do is to find ways to positively change the negative aspects of your life—a bad job or relationship. Doing so will help you brighten your attitude—and improve your chances of living longer.

Stress

 Understand the effects of stress on your body.

Once upon a time, we had to stand up to saber-toothed tigers and flee from other primeval dangers. We developed a protective "fight or flight" reaction. Now, however, if we get cut off in traffic or receive bad news, the same mechanism takes hold. Our heart races, our blood pressure rises, and our muscles tighten up. Our senses become sharper, and we feel nervous, apprehensive, and tense. This happens because the brain is releasing the stress hormones cortisol, epinephrine (adrenaline), and norepinephrine into our blood. They regulate the changes that carry extra sugar and fatty acids to the brain and muscles for fuel and constrict the blood vessels that supply less vital areas such as the skin and stomach.

When this reaction is ongoing, the body can be seriously affected. Some of the effects are relatively minor, such as stomach upset or sleeplessness, while at the same time, others may impact your longevity, causing heart disease, diabetes, and a poorly functioning immune system. Here are some examples.

Increased blood pressure. At least 20 studies that looked at bus drivers in various cities—a stressful job with high demands but little sense of control—have found that they had higher rates of mortality from heart disease. And a study in the journal *Stroke* showed that middle-aged women who have major increases in blood pressure due to stress have an increased risk of stroke.

Increased cholesterol levels. In a study of certified public accountants, cholesterol levels were measured from January to the April 15 tax deadline. The accountants had as much as a 100 mg/dL increase in their cholesterol during that highly stressful time. High cholesterol levels can lead to atherosclerosis, which increases the risk of heart attack and stroke.

Increased risk of ischemia (impaired blood flow to the heart). The Ischemic Heart Disease Life Stress Monitoring Program assigned heart attack patients to a behavior modification group or a control group. One year later, the death rate for the group that changed behavior was half that of the group that didn't change its behavior. Seven years later, the behavior modification group was less likely to have had additional heart attacks.

Reduced immunity. People under stress have lower levels of the natural killer cells that fight tumors and infection and of the T cells that switch on the immune response. Studies have shown greater numbers of colds in college students during exam periods and decreased immune system function—including more colds—in people caring for seriously ill spouses.

Stress has also been found to increase the incidence of these dangerous conditions.

Diabetes. Stress can increase blood sugar and suppress insulin, which regulates blood sugar levels, thereby raising the risk of diabetes, and, possibly, its own set of attendant problems.

Depression. Stress can produce depression.

Asthma. Stress can worsen asthma.

Researchers reporting in the *New England Journal of Medicine* identify these six major indicators of stress.

- High blood pressure
- Weakened immunity
- Weakened muscles
- Bone loss
- Increase in blood sugar
- Increase in cholesterol levels

Once you recognize these symptoms, look for an ongoing stressor that is causing the unhealthy conditions. Then try to eliminate or reduce it.

 Find alternative ways to fight stress.

Western medicine is just starting to take a look at the alternative therapies that have been calming minds for centuries all over the world, including Asia, Europe, and Latin America. You can use them to still the stress that can slow down your century-long journey.

A large body of evidence shows that relaxation strategies, including meditation, biofeedback, and yoga, are effective in reducing stress. They reduce heart rate, slow breathing, increase alpha brain waves (which are produced when you are relaxed), and clear the mind of harmful thoughts. The chart on page 108 outlines several effective ways to beat the stress that can be taking a toll on your body.

 ## Let a pet be your therapist.

Just one look at those big brown eyes staring adoringly at you and the cares of the day melt away. Pets have a positive effect on your immune system because they help alleviate dangerous stress—and simply add to your enjoyment of life. It doesn't matter whether your pet is a pedigree, a mutt, or an alley cat. Even a hamster, guinea pig, or bird can help you live longer.

Several studies support the connection between pets and better health. When researchers at Johns Hopkins Medical Center followed up on patients a year after a heart attack, they found that 50 out of 53 people with pets were alive compared with 17 of 39 who weren't pet owners. It's also been shown that people undergoing psychotherapy or recovering from illnesses are healthier when pets are around.

Pets have also been shown to help lower blood pressure. And they give people another reason to stay alive and healthy.

 ## Exercise away stress.

After as few as 10 to 20 minutes of intense aerobic exercise—the sustained kind that gets your heart beating faster—the brain releases epinephrine, which gives us a surge of energy, and endorphins, the "feel-good" hormones, into your system. You begin to breathe more deeply, thus moving more oxygen to muscles that were being short-changed during a stress reaction. Then lactic acid, cellular waste that is a major muscle irritant, begins to be removed from your body.

(continued on page 110)

Stress Reduction Techniques

TECHNIQUE	DEFINITION	PROCEDURES
Relaxation Strategies		
Biofeedback	Conscious control of involuntary body functions through concentration	Ele⁀odes are attached to the body to measure muscular tension, heart rate, and temerature. A high-pitched sound from the monitor indicates stress, teaching you how to recognize your body's stress signals. The pitch becomes lower as you consciously relax, slowing your breathing and heart rate and releasing muscle tension.
Meditation	Concentration on one object	A number of meditation practices exist, from yoga to transcendental meditation and self-hypnosis. These techniques generally involve sitting or lying comfortably, closing your eyes, and silently repeating and focusing on a one-syllable word, or mantra, to prevent distraction and promote relaxation.
Relaxation Response	Natural state of self-induced relaxation, introduced by Herbert Benson, M.D.	Conscious thoughts are blocked using any of a variety of strategies that employ four elements: a mental device on which to focus to enhance concentration; a passive attitude; a comfortable, relaxed position; and a quiet environment. Strategies to achieve the relaxation response include deep breathing, progressive muscle relaxation, meditation, aromatherapy, and biofeedback.
Mind-Body Intervention		
Hypnosis	Procedure in which a therapist initiates a relaxation response and helps divert attention away from everyday activities and into ways of addressing a problem	The hypnotherapist initiates a relaxation response, helps you shift your thoughts away from everyday life, then asks you to imagine that you are experiencing a situation that causes stress and are responding in a relaxed manner. After several sessions, you should be able to translate the rehearsed mental image into real-life behavior.

TECHNIQUE	DEFINITION	PROCEDURES
Complementary Therapies		
Acupressure	Ancient Chinese healing technique based on the idea that good health results from a balanced flow of chi, the vital organizing force of the body, which flows along paths known as meridians. It is believed that if the flow of chi is interrupted or blocked, illness and disease set in. Acupressure uses the application of pressure to correct blockages along meridians.	Fingers press key points on the surface of the skin to stimulate the body's natural healing abilities. The pressure is thought to release muscular tension and improve circulation.
Acupuncture	Ancient Chinese healing technique based on the idea that good health results from a balanced flow of chi (see acupressure elsewhere in this chart). Acupuncture uses the insertion of small needles into the skin to correct blockages along meridians.	Thin needles are inserted just below the skin at key points to stimulate the body's natural healing abilities. Studies indicate that acupuncture releases endorphins, hormones that counteract pain and diminish the effect of stress hormones.
Meditative Movement Therapies		
Tai chi	Meditative and physical exercise designed to promote physical strength, mental clarity, and emotional serenity	Tai chi uses flowing body movements—much like modern dance in slow motion—to generate and feel energy throughout the body and promote better mental and physical health.
Yoga	Series of complex stretching exercises combined with deep breathing, meditation, and postures. It is thought to restore harmony and balance between the body and soul.	Yoga involves the regular practice of various postures and exercises, often along with meditation. It can lower blood pressure and increase the body's strength and flexibility.

Studies show that exercise works. A study at California State University found that a 10-minute walk could provide a positive mental outlook for as long as two hours afterward. A report issued by the Surgeon General points out that regular physical activity reduces the symptoms of anxiety and depression.

To get health benefits, try aerobic exercise such as walking, jogging, or running. Swimming, with its sensation of reconnecting to the womb or even our primordial beginnings, is a soothing way to eliminate stress. Ballroom dancing is enjoying a renaissance as people waltz their way through a stress-relieving combination of exercise, music, and companionship.

■ APPENDIX
Suggested Resources

Books

Inlander, Charles B. and Michael A. Donio. *Medicare Made Easy.* Allentown, Pa.: People's Medical Society, 1999.

Inlander, Charles B. and Cynthia K. Moran. *Stress: 63 Ways to Relieve Tension and Stay Healthy.* New York: Walker, 1996.

Inlander, Charles B. and Eugene Pavalon. *Your Medical Rights.* Allentown, Pa.: People's Medical Society, 1994.

Khanna, Vikram, M.H.S. *Managed Care Made Easy.* Allentown, Pa.: People's Medical Society, 1997.

Organizations

American Association of Retired Persons
601 E. St., NW
Washington, DC 20049
800-424-3410
www.aarp.org

American Cancer Society
1599 Clifton Rd., NE
Atlanta, GA 303329-4251
404-320-3333
800-227-2345
www.cancer.org

American Diabetes Association
National Center
1660 Duke St.
Alexandria, VA 22314
703-549-1500
800-342-2383
www.diabetes.org

American Heart Association
7272 Greenville Ave.
Dallas, TX 75231-4596
214-373-6300
800-242-8721
www.americanheart.org

American Hospital Association
1 N. Franklin St., Suite 2700
Chicago, IL 60606
312-422-3000
www.aha.org

American Lung Association
1740 Broadway, 14th Floor
New York, NY 10019-4374
212-315-8700
800-586-4872
www.lungusa.org

People's Medical Society
462 Walnut St.
Allentown, PA 18102
610-770-1670
www.peoplesmed.org

■ INDEX